The Eating Addiction Relapse Prevention Workbook

**For Compulsive Overeaters,
Binge Eaters, and Food Addicts**

Developed by
Dr. Stephen F. Grinstead and
Dr. Shari Stillman-Corbitt

Based in Part on the Gorski-CENAPS® Model

© 2008 Stephen F. Grinstead
Printed in the United States of America

Additional copies are available from the publisher:
  Herald House/Independence Press
  1001 West Walnut
  P.O. Box 390
  Independence, MO 64051-0390
  Phone: 1-800-767-8181 or (816) 521-3015
  Fax: (816) 521-3066
  Web site: *www.relapse.org*

For training contact:
  The CENAPS Corporation
  6147 Deltona Blvd.
  Spring Hill, FL 34606
  Phone: (352) 596-8000
  Fax: (352) 596-8002
  E-mail: *info@cenaps.com*

ISBN: 978-0-8309-1407-4

Contents

Acknowledgments 5

Dr. Grinstead's Comments 5

Dr. Stillman-Corbitt's Comments 5

Goals of This Workbook 6

Exercise 1: Creating Your Healthy Living Plan 10

Part 1: Principles of a Healthy Living Plan 10

    Personalizing Your Own Healthy Living Plan 10

Part 2: Defining Abstinence for You 11

Part 3: Biological Aspects of Eating Addiction 12

    Common Trigger Foods 12

    Responses to the Biological or Physical Aspects of Eating Addiction 12

Part 4: Psychological Aspects of Eating Addiction 13

    Common Thoughts That Trigger Cravings 13

    Common Feelings That Emerge When Not "Pushed Down" or "Swallowed"
        with Eating 13

Part 5: Behavioral Aspects of Eating Addiction 14

    Eating Behaviors That Trigger Eating Addiction 14

Part 6: Social Aspects of Eating Addiction 15

    Social Conditions That Trigger Eating Addiction 15

Part 7: Spiritual Aspects of Eating Addiction 17

Part 8: Preliminary Healthy Living Plan 18

    Biological Plan 18

    Psychological Plan 19

    Social Plan 19

    Spiritual Plan 20

Exercise 2: Creating Your Personalized Definition of Abstinence 21

Part 1: What Is Abstinence? 21

Part 2: Developing Your Personalized Definition 21

Part 3: Finalizing Your Personalized Definition of Abstinence 22

Part 4: Your Definition of Abstinence Summary 23

Exercise 3: Eating Addiction Problem Checklist 24

Part 1: Interpreting the Eating Addiction Problem Checklist 26

Part 2: Eating Addiction Problem Checklist Summary 27

Exercise 4: Decision Making 28

Part 1: What You Wanted 28

Part 2: What You Learned 29

Part 3: The Decision to Stop Using Eating as a Coping Tool 29

    The Benefits and Disadvantages of Eating Compulsively/Addictively 30

Part 4: Decision Making Summary 31

Exercise 5: Intervention Planning **32**

Part 1: Craving Intervention Planning 32

Part 2: Relapse Intervention Planning 34

Part 3: The Intervention Plan Summary 36

Exercise 6: The Healthy Living Contract **37**

Part 1: Presenting Problems 37

Part 2: Presenting Problem Summary 39

Part 3: Completing the Healthy Living Contract 40

Part 4: The Healthy Living Contract Summary 42

Exercise 7: High-Risk Situations **43**

Part 1: Identifying High-Risk Situations 43

Part 2: The Eating Addiction High-Risk Situation List 45

Part 3: High-Risk Situation Summary Discussion Questions 49

Exercise 8: Situation Mapping **51**

Part 1: Mapping an Ineffectively Managed Situation 51

Part 2: Mapping an Effectively Managed Situation 54

Part 3: Mapping a Future High-Risk Situation 57

Part 4: Situation Mapping Summary 61

Exercise 9: Managing High-Risk Situations **62**

Part 1: Managing Thoughts 65

Part 2: Managing Feelings 66

Part 3: Managing Urges 70

Part 4: Managing Actions/Behaviors 71

Part 5: Tying It All Together 73

Part 6: High-Risk Situation Management Summary 76

Exercise 10: Recovery Planning **77**

Part 1: Selecting Recovery Activities 77

Part 2: The Schedule of Recovery Activities 84

Part 3: Testing the Schedule of Recovery Activities 86

Part 4: Recovery Planning Summary 88

Exercise 11: Final Evaluation **89**

A Final Word **91**

Acknowledgments

Dr. Grinstead's Comments

There are several people that deserve special acknowledgment for making this workbook possible. First, there is *Terence T. Gorski*, founder and president of The Gorski-CENAPS® Corporation, who helped me develop and publish the *Food Addiction Workbook* this book is based on. I want to especially thank *Dr. Shari Stillman-Corbitt*, a colleague I finally found after many years of searching, who helped me improve the original work and bring it to its final form. Dr. Corbitt has extensive education and experience in working with patients with eating disorders including eating addiction.

I want to extend my thanks to *Kay Holmes* and *Gabrielle Antolovich* who helped develop several exercises in that first workbook, including the *Healthy Living Plan* and the *High-Risk Situation List*. They also helped modify the original *Food Problem Checklist* exercise that we have modified again and given a new title: *Eating Addiction Problem Checklist*.

I also want to thank *Ellen Gruber-Grinstead*, my wife and partner in life as well as business, for her assistance in analyzing, editing, and formatting this book (and also the original *Food Addiction Recovery and Relapse Prevention Workbook*) and her encouragement and emotional support the past twenty years. And finally I want to especially thank my private-practice clients who helped me personally field-test many of the exercises in these two workbooks.

—*Stephen F. Grinstead, Dr. AD, LMFT, ACRPS, CADC-II*

Dr. Stillman-Corbitt's Comments

There are so many people I would like to thank who have supported me to the place where I can now contribute to this publication in a meaningful way. My deepest gratitude goes to my husband for his unflagging support, love, and encouragement. I would also like to thank the extraordinary and wise women who have taught me all I ever needed to know: *Donna Siegmann, JoAnn Alexander, Nancy Jarrell, Lynn Sucher, Elaine Alexander, and Jackie Katz*.

I would also like to thank all of my colleagues at Sierra Tucson who make every day a distinct pleasure. Finally, I would like to make a special acknowledgement to *Becky Jackson*, author of *Dieting, a Dry Drunk*, and her Web site *www.dietingrecovery.com*. Becky's expertise in this field serves as the foundation for my knowledge, and areas of this book where I draw from her work have been noted accordingly. Becky—my most heartfelt thanks.

—*Shari Stillman-Corbitt, Psy.D.*

Goals of This Workbook

This workbook is for compulsive overeaters, food addicts, and binge eaters. These terms describe people who use eating and food to manage feelings and cope with life. Although the primary purpose of this workbook is to help you develop a relapse prevention plan and create a schedule of activities to assist in that goal, we believe you must first develop a definition of abstinence that works for you and an effective recovery plan that is life enhancing, which we refer to in this workbook as a Healthy Living Plan. Therefore, the first five exercises in this book are designed to take you through a series of steps to make sure that you are stable in your recovery. Some of you may already be working a solid recovery program, but we believe these exercises can also benefit you.

- **Exercise 1:** Looking at the principles of a Healthy Living Plan from a biopsychosocial-spiritual perspective, then listing your personal *triggers* in each of those categories and creating your own Healthy Living Plan.

- **Exercise 2:** Learning how to develop your personalized definition of abstinence as an important component of your recovery and Healthy Living Plan.

- **Exercise 3:** Completing the *Eating Addiction Problem Checklist* to help determine your level of problem (past and/or present) with compulsive use of eating.

- **Exercise 4:** Looking at the pros and cons concerning the way you have used eating in the past and making a decision to stop using eating as a coping tool.

- **Exercise 5:** Creating a craving management plan and an early relapse intervention plan designed to help you avoid relapse in the early stages of your recovery.

- **Exercise 6:** Looking at your presenting problems with eating and personalizing your own *Healthy Living Contract.*

The last five exercises in this book help you identify and manage high-risk situations that could set you up for relapse despite your commitment to your *Healthy Living Plan* (recovery) and develop an effective recovery plan designed to help you manage those high-risk situations.

- **Exercise 7:** Defining high-risk situations and picking your own personal high-risk situation that you would like to learn to manage.

- **Exercise 8:** Mapping (exploring) past ineffectively managed and effectively managed high-risk situations, then using that information to project and explore a future high-risk situation.

- **Exercise 9:** Learning to identify and manage personal reactions to high-risk situations by exploring your automatic thinking, feelings, urges, actions, and social reactions that drive the relapse process and are triggered when you encounter a high-risk situation.

- **Exercise 10:** Developing a personalized recovery plan by selecting and scheduling recovery activities that will help you identify and manage future high-risk situations.

- **Exercise 11:** Completing a final evaluation process that asks you to complete a checklist to determine how well you believe you did completing this workbook.

Some of you may be a normal weight, if your metabolism is such that you don't gain weight, or some of you may purge calories through excessive exercise. However, many of you will probably be overweight, or "see-sawing" up and down, as you try first one magic pill, diet, or program, and then another. Some of you may be obese—the definition of which states you are more than 20 percent over the weight suggested by actuarial tables. You may know that you are destroying and distorting your body, but may be unable to stop eating compulsively.

There are several variations of eating disorders listed in the DSM IV (*Diagnostic and Statistical Manual of Mental Disorders*, fourth edition). Anorexia nervosa (compulsive starving) and bulimia nervosa—purging type (bingeing and then getting rid of the food by vomiting, laxative abuse, diuretics, intermittent food restriction, or excessive exercise) are also serious conditions, but they are *not* the subjects of this workbook. They have been given a great deal of medical attention because they are complex psychiatric disorders and can quickly become life threatening. The compulsive overeater is described in the DSM simply as a "nonpurging bulimic" and has traditionally been viewed as weak willed. This describes those of us who *binge* or eat food in larger amounts than is needed for fuel, but do not immediately get rid of it. Or we may not binge in large quantities but graze throughout the bulk of each day, never allowing ourselves to feel physical hunger. There is a section of the DSM that indicates where more research is needed. In that area is a *binge-eating disorder* that more accurately matches the compulsive/addictive eating pattern for which this workbook is written. The newly revised DSM-IV-TR does not include a diagnostic category for binge-eating disorder, but perhaps in the next edition of the DSM this subject will receive the attention it deserves. In the meantime, the problem still exists.

> **Compulsive overeaters use eating to
> manage feelings and cope with life.**

This workbook, and the research that went into it, was written to offer hope to those who use eating to avoid feelings and cope with life. We do not address the anorexia or bulimia, but focus only on compulsive or addictive overeating. Our goal is to help you define your abstinence and find tools for living so that excess eating will no longer be needed to numb, medicate, or push down feelings. This workbook is not a "one size fits all." It is more of a road map and certainly not a straitjacket. It was designed to help you create an individualized, highly personalized recovery plan. For this workbook to be effective, you need to determine whether or not you have a compulsive/addictive eating problem. Those who have crossed the line and no longer have predictable control of their eating, even when it is harmful to them in some way, have an addiction/compulsion to eat. We are speaking here of the most simple description of addiction: the continued use of a mood-altering substance or behavior, despite negative consequences. The consequences may be physical, emotional, social, interrelational, legal, spiritual, or personal (as in shame or poor esteem).

Some people with eating problems have dealt with other addictions (alcohol/other drugs) and report it to be more difficult when they try to use identical tools in dealing with compulsive/addictive eating. There are many similarities, no matter what chemical or behavior is being used to mood alter or change feelings. Alcoholics, for instance, don't stop drinking all fluids, only alcoholic fluids. Similarly, eating addicts in recovery don't stop eating all foods, but do abstain from their compulsive or other unhealthy eating behaviors and eat highly nutritional, nourishing foods needed for health and well-being.

In eating addiction recovery, many have found it is critically important to abstain from addictive behaviors around eating. This means changing basic eating behaviors or eating patterns that support compulsive overeating, such as abstaining from gobbling, eating all the time rather than only at meal times, eating while driving, standing, etc. This is similar to alcoholics in recovery being told to stay away from drinking juice in a wineglass or non-alcoholic beers in a bar to avoid being "triggered" to drink alcohol. Likewise, some alcoholics in recovery have found the tinkling of ice in a glass can bring on urges for alcohol and are encouraged not to use ice in drinks to distract themselves from their recovery. These suggestions help addicts avoid the triggering of cravings and possible relapse. Addictive behaviors around eating can also trigger relapse. This is why compulsive overeaters find it helpful to be mindful of not just what they eat (a healthy meal plan), but also how they eat (healthy eating patterns), when they eat (a healthy meal schedule), and how much they eat (healthy portion control). Getting clear on what, how, how much, and how often you eat will make your recovery process smoother with less cravings. It will also reduce your incidence and length of relapse.

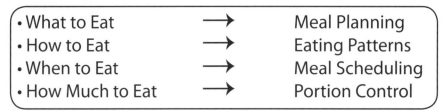

• What to Eat	→	Meal Planning
• How to Eat	→	Eating Patterns
• When to Eat	→	Meal Scheduling
• How Much to Eat	→	Portion Control

This workbook is *not* another diet book. Knowing what to eat and how to eat can be learned through your medical provider, a nutritionist or registered dietician, or any of the many books available. Likewise, we do not want to discuss biochemistry (though we know it is important) or differences in metabolism and nutritional needs. This workbook is designed to assist you in discovering and understanding your personal *relapse triggers* whether they are in response to specific foods, particular experiences, or certain feelings. We call these *high-risk situations* (HRS). Not recognizing or ignoring these situations puts you at greater risk for relapse. You will create a definition of abstinence for yourself—your sober pattern of eating that will support you in avoiding random or spontaneous eating behaviors. Finally, you will also create a *Healthy Living Plan*, which will outline the necessary ingredients for your recovery. Because this plan is individualized, you will develop a personalized *Craving Management Plan* and *Relapse Intervention Plan*. This will require you to involve trusted others, who have been told (by you) what to look for and how to intervene, should they see behaviors you have described as high risk.

To fully utilize the tools in this workbook, you will need to do more than just read and complete the exercises. You will need to discuss your responses with someone who can help you sort out the thoughts and feelings that inevitably come up as a result of the self-examination required. You cannot do this alone. You will need to work with someone who understands the relapse process and also knows eating disorders. They need to understand that this is *your* journey, *your* exploration, and as such will be highly personal. It will probably not look like anyone else's program, although they may have common themes. This helper could be a sponsor, counselor, therapist, nutritionist, or friend. It is possible to do these exercises as a group process, with a qualified facilitator. As long as everyone is committed to individual exploration and discovery, it works very well. We suggest you avoid those who have an absolute idea of what your program *should* look like. Rather, it is important that the person you choose to share your journey with be someone who can respect your ability to develop, over time, a workable program for *you*. This will be a program you can live with, not follow for a brief time (like a diet) and then abandon. Things we suggest you look for in a person are

1. eating disorder knowledge and experience, especially in compulsive/binge/addictive eating;

2. relapse prevention training and experience;

3. a trustworthy person with whom you are willing to be *absolutely honest*; and

4. a person who can be honest, direct, and compassionate with you.

Remember:

- **compassion without honesty is enabling;**
- **honesty without compassion is brutality.**

Go to the next page and start *Exerise 1: Creating Your Healthy Living Plan.*

Exercise 1: Creating Your Healthy Living Plan

Part 1: Principles of a Healthy Living Plan

Eating Addiction/compulsion is a biopsychosocialspiritual phenomenon. The four different aspects of the disease mean there are several components to consider.

The *bio* (biological or physical) aspect deals with the body—weight, diet, exercise, and illness issues.

The *psycho* (psychological or emotional) aspect deals with what you believe and how you think about eating and the use of eating to change how you feel. These are automatic habitual behaviors that lock you into patterns of compulsive overeating. You may experience mood swings, depression, and/or anger. You may also experience emotional distance from yourself and others due to your overeating. In some cases, self-consciousness about your weight may bring up feelings of loneliness or separation/isolation.

The *social* aspect deals with your relationship to eating and people. For instance, giving yourself permission to only be with people who eat like you eat, or at least are not critical of your eating, can isolate you. The social aspect also looks at your relationship to yourself in the world.

The *spiritual* aspect deals with your connection to yourself, others, and a Higher Power or universal order. Part of this connection may show up as an enthusiasm for life.

Personalizing Your Own Healthy Living Plan

The Endless Search for the Right Diet

Some people only want to find the right diet and lose weight, concentrating only on the (bio) body. Experience and research has shown us that diets do not work as long-term solutions for people addicted to eating. In fact, diets can become part of the addictive process and may cause physical problems within the body. The desperate search for another diet, exercise, or eating solution continues and becomes part of a reinforcing process. See if this sounds familiar when starting a new diet:

1.   Excitement—this one will work!!

2.   Some success—now I'm OK.

3.   Growing discouragement/deprivation—I'm tired of this.

4.   Bingeing or overeating—I've failed.

5.   Discouragement and depression—why try?

6.   The search continues for a new diet—the cycle begins again.

When you look at the phases of a new diet, it is clear that the first two parts feel powerful, but are followed by a growing feeling of "I can't have something vital that I need and want" (deprivation) and "this can't work, it's hopeless and I'm helpless" (discouragement). Any one approach (bio-psycho-social-spiritual) alone is not enough, but, if these four are combined, they are a powerful response to addictive/compulsive eating.

10

Looking for the Magical Psycho-Spiritual Solution

Others look for (psychological) emotional solutions, believing that Twelve-Step programs, therapy, or turning to friends and partners will solve their compulsive overeating. Dealing with feelings while continuing to use compulsive eating behaviors has not stopped their eating addiction. Likewise, while being helpful, concentrating on the spiritual, such as only turning to God (without a recovery process), has not served most people in dealing with their eating compulsions in the long term.

Developing a Biopsychosocialspiritual Approach

To truly deal with this complex issue of eating addiction/compulsion, we must approach it with a personalized multilayered biopsychosocialspiritual recovery process. We can never forget the eating issues, but must keep in mind the many levels of addiction and recovery.

As part of your Healthy Living Plan you will need to choose a number of activities to deal with the various aspects of your eating compulsion/addiction. We will offer you some possibilities in each of the biopsychosocialspiritual areas to support you in developing your personal plan. We strongly encourage you to not do this alone, but to seek help from qualified people such as certified nutritionists for meal planning and an exercise specialist working in collaboration with your doctor. Your plan will probably change or evolve over time, but it is important to make some decisions, commit to those decisions, and follow them through. Making a commitment to a plan, and then sticking to it, is a way to confront the ongoing onslaught of your addiction/compulsion. *What are you willing to do—beginning now?*

Part 2: Defining Abstinence for You

It is critically important for the foundation of your Healthy Living Plan that you develop *a definition of abstinence* that works for you as your "sobriety." Just as the recovering alcoholic strives to live in as healthy a manner as possible, the bottom line is not drinking alcohol. So, too, the recovering compulsive overeater needs a bottom-line definition of sobriety or abstinence from their eating addiction. Your definition should be personalized to the problematic behaviors that have plagued you in your illness.

If you have been a compulsive grazer, eating small portions practically nonstop throughout your day, examples of this definition might sound like, "I eat moderate portions during planned and balanced meals five times per day," or three times per day, or whatever number of meals feels right for your lifestyle. If you have not been a breakfast eater, but ate an enormous lunch and dinner, your definition may sound like, "I eat three moderate and balanced meals daily and I don't skip meals." Work with your medical provider, registered dietician, or nutritionist to determine what number of meals you should be eating each day.

This is not a definition that should get revamped on a daily basis, but should be a bottom line that can be adhered to as a regular course of living. Many recovering compulsive overeaters have shared great fear about "restricting" the number of times they will be "allowed" to eat daily.

Remember—This Is Not a Diet!

You are going to successfully learn how to abstain from compulsive overeating; many recovering alcoholics felt fear about how they would abstain from alcohol. It is natural and normal that you may have some fears, as well, about removing excessive eating from your life. You will need to develop a support team to help you get on track and remain abstinent. You will learn more about this in *Exercise 2*, as well as seeing how you can create your own definition of abstinence.

Go to Part 3 to explore the
Biological Aspects of Eating Addiction

Part 3: Biological Aspects of Eating Addiction

Common Trigger Foods

Trigger foods make you want to eat more of either that food or any food. Here are some of the more common trigger foods:

1. Refined sugars

2. Chocolate

3. Refined flours

4. High-fat processed foods

5. High-salt processed foods

6. Fried foods

List yours here:

_____   _____

_____   _____

_____   _____

List the trigger foods you are willing to eliminate from your food plan for now:

_____   _____

_____   _____

_____   _____

Responses to the Biological or Physical Aspects of Eating Addiction

1. Develop a healthy eating plan you can stick to for a period of time. It may only be for a few days, but you will commit to it completely. You should see a certified nutritionist or doctor to develop this plan.

2. Develop an exercise plan that works for your body and your present health condition, avoiding doing too much, too fast. *Remember, easy does it, but do it!* It is important to seek medical advice when developing this plan.

3. Write out your plan, sign it, and share it with your sponsor or therapist. This will help strengthen your commitment to your plan.

The real point is to start now, not tomorrow. What are you willing to do for your recovery right now? Your choices will continue to be modified as you grow and develop in your recovery process. What are you willing to do, right now, for a specified period of time? At the end of this exercise you will be asked to develop your own personal biopsychosocial-spiritual Healthy Living Plan.

> **Go to Part 4 to explore the**
> **Psychological Aspects of Eating Addiction.**

Part 4: Psychological Aspects of Eating Addiction

Common Thoughts That Trigger Cravings

A question for you to consider: *Does irrational thinking lead to cravings?*

Remember that old automatic patterns of thinking can lead to obsessing or craving about using eating compulsively.

1. I'm starving to death.

2. This is way too hard to avoid.

3. Just this once won't hurt me.

4. I'll stay in control this time.

5. I deserve a reward.

6. I'd feel better if I could only eat some _____.

7. I didn't eat breakfast; I need to catch up.

8. My next diet will do it—tomorrow.

9. I have a thyroid or other glandular or genetic problem—not an eating problem.

10. The world is *fataphobic*, so I won't worry about my weight.

11. Being overweight runs in my family, and they all eat like me.

List your personal automatic thoughts here:

_____   _____

_____   _____

_____   _____

If you can identify and challenge these preprogrammed messages and replace them with healthier ways of thinking, you can avoid the pain of compulsive overeating. You will get a chance to challenge this type of thinking later in the workbook.

Common Feelings That Emerge When Not "Pushed Down" or "Swallowed" with Eating

Another question for you to consider: *Does every feeling you have translate to hunger?*

If you suppress your feelings immediately with food, you'll never know what those feelings are. If you abstain from compulsive overeating when feelings come up, you can observe them, name them, share about them, and let them go. Below are two different groups of feelings. The first is a feeling checklist with a rating scale, and the second is a list of twelve feelings. Look these over and think about the feelings you attempt to cover with compulsive overeating, then record your feelings in the space indicated below.

- **Feeling Checklist**

❑ Strong	or	❑ Weak?	How strong is the feeling? (0–10) _____
❑ Angry	or	❑ Caring?	How strong is the feeling? (0–10) _____
❑ Happy	or	❑ Sad?	How strong is the feeling? (0–10) _____
❑ Safe	or	❑ Threatened?	How strong is the feeling? (0–10) _____
❑ Fulfilled	or	❑ Frustrated?	How strong is the feeling? (0–10) _____
❑ Connected	or	❑ Lonely?	How strong is the feeling? (0–10) _____
❑ Proud	or	❑ Ashamed?	How strong is the feeling? (0–10) _____
❑ Peaceful	or	❑ Agitated?	How strong is the feeling? (0–10) _____

- **List of Feelings**

1. Anger	2. Rage	3. Sexual desire	4. Joy
5. Hurt	6. Loneliness	7. Inadequacy	8. Shame
9. Passion	10. Fear	11. Self-esteem/pride in self	12. Excitement

List your feelings here:

_____   _____

_____   _____

_____   _____

After you have identified the feeling and talked about it, the hunger (or the translation of that feeling to hunger) may disappear. In a later exercise you will develop an effective feeling management plan.

> **Go to Part 5 to explore the**
> **Behavioral Aspects of Eating Addiction.**

Part 5: Behavioral Aspects of Eating Addiction

Eating Behaviors That Trigger Eating Addiction

1. Gobbling

2. Eating whatever is at hand

3. Eating food that's free or extra at buffets because it is available and "nobody will notice"

4. Not eating enough and having hunger overwhelm you later

5. Eating too much of any food

6. Eating to the point of being too full

7. Sneaking, hiding, stealing food

8. Hanging out with your binge buddies, that is, letting others coax, con, push you into eating like them when it is not in your best interest

14

9. Eating at times when you did not plan to, because you didn't take the time to make your healthy eating plan or didn't have the right food available when you needed it

10. Eating whenever you want, all day long—*grazing*

11. Eating while standing, moving about, on the run, driving, on the phone, watching TV

12. Eating late at night

13. Eating without realizing that you've eaten

14. Finishing what's on your plate because you grew up in a family with a "clean-plate club"

List your trigger behaviors here:

_____   _____

_____   _____

_____   _____

> **Go to Part 6 to explore the
> Social Aspects of Eating Addiction.**

Part 6: Social Aspects of Eating Addiction

We often try to talk ourselves out of taking immediate action to solve the problems we ate our way into, such as "I'll go on that new diet next week" or "I'll start exercising tomorrow." We try to rationalize our way out of our eating addiction. We make unrealistic promises to ourselves while we continue to compulsively overeat. However, when faced with the reality of our situation through family or friends, we feel ashamed and often stuff those feelings down. Some common social triggers (at work; with friends, intimate partners, parents, and children) are listed below.

Social Conditions That Trigger Eating Addiction

1. My wife/husband/partner criticizes me.

2. My job is too hard for me and nobody likes me.

3. My mother/father criticizes me.

4. My children are ashamed of me.

5. Airline travel is very difficult for me.

List your social triggers here:

_____   _____

_____   _____

_____   _____

We can also develop *magical thinking* about what our relationships will look like when we have lost weight. We often believe that just losing weight will solve all of our relationship problems. This just isn't true. Losing weight will make you thinner; it won't solve any other problems. To solve other problems you have to set up a problem-solving plan. These unrealistic fantasies or expectations about how being thin will fix your relationships can act as a relapse trigger. The belief that losing weight will automatically repair our relationship

15

problems can drive us into compulsive dieting and then set us up for disillusionment when we get thin and still have dysfunctional relationships.

List three of your most important relationships below and identify the problems that you believe losing weight will automatically and magically fix.

1. Relationship #1: _____

    Problems I believe losing weight will solve: _____

    _____

2. Relationship #2: _____

    Problems I believe losing weight will solve: _____

    _____

3. Relationship #3: _____

    Problems I believe losing weight will solve: _____

    _____

**Go to Part 7 to explore the
Spiritual Aspects of Eating Addiction.**

Part 7: Spiritual Aspects of Eating Addiction

We want to begin this section by differentiating between the terms "spiritual" and "religious." By *spiritual*, we mean a feeling of being connected; a right to be here and take up space on the planet; a feeling of having a purpose, being part of the real world, or being part of a greater whole. By *religious*, we mean an organized body of beliefs and rules usually congregating at a church, synagogue, or other place of worship.

Some people find it easy to ask God for help, even regarding an eating addiction. Others, however, need to think of G.O.D. as Good Orderly Direction, a Healthy Eating Plan, and appropriate support people who understand eating addiction.

Many eating-addicted people feel their spirit is trapped inside their body, starving for connection. Getting thin, they have found, does not necessarily release their trapped spirit. It may release stored feelings, such as resentments, anger, frustration, disappointment, sexual desires, shame, or self-hatred that need to be dealt with. If they aren't, these feelings often trigger discomfort that many of us experience as hunger. The new thin person starts yet another bout of eating compulsively/addictively to deal with the emotional discomfort, and the addictive cycle continues.

It is important to think about the disease of eating addiction as being a multilayered problem that needs a comprehensive recovery plan. This may include attending specific self-help meetings, such as Overeaters Anonymous and other support available through eating addiction treatment facilities, therapists, counselors, churches, or other organizations. Group participation can help you feel less alone and disconnected.

1. Is there a higher meaning or purpose to your life? ❏ Yes ❏ No ❏ Unsure

    Please explain: _____

    _____

2. How has your eating addiction affected your sense of meaning and purpose in life?

    _____

    _____

3. Do you have a personal relationship with God or some Higher Power that gives you courage, strength, and hope? ❏ Yes ❏ No ❏ Unsure

    Please explain: _____

    _____

4. How has your eating addiction affected your relationship with your Higher Power?

    Please explain: _____

    _____

5. Do you have a spiritual program of recovery? ❏ Yes ❏ No ❏ Unsure

    Please explain: _____

    _____

Let's take a moment to summarize what we have discussed so far. Compulsive overeating and yo-yoing between weight-gain/weight-loss dampens the spirit and enthusiasm for life. Regulating your life with an eating plan can help you emotionally stabilize after the first three to four weeks. During the first few days of a new eating plan, the emotions will probably feel more reactive, since we are no longer using eating to comfort, cope, or sedate. Using some of the suggested tools in the emotional (psycho) recovery list can help you through these times. This can make it easier to get (back) into the life you are meant to live.

Just because the world is fataphobic, and I'm required to "do lunch" and go to banquets for my job, doesn't mean I have to participate. Just because my family and social life is riddled with compulsive overeaters and our activities up until now have been eating-focused, doesn't mean I have to continue to participate.

Remember, it is difficult to get sober from alcohol in a bar while still hanging out with your old bar buddies. Likewise it is difficult to become abstinent from eating addiction while still participating in eating-focused rituals with your old binge buddies or enabling family members. It doesn't mean *never* seeing your old friends again, although it may mean developing a different relationship with them, such as spending time talking together rather than eating together.

Recovery from eating addiction means setting new boundaries and developing a support network that enhances your recovery process and the new relationships with the people in your life. Creating a new support network is essential for long-term recovery from eating addiction. You deserve this support!

By using what you have learned in this exercise you now have a chance to develop a preliminary Healthy Living (recovery) Plan that focuses on all four of the biopsychosocial-spiritual areas covered earlier.

> **Go to Part 8 and complete your Preliminary Healthy Living Plan.**

Part 8: Preliminary Healthy Living Plan

INSTRUCTIONS: Before your next group or individual session, take a few minutes to develop your own personal biopsychosocialspiritual Healthy Living Plan—remember, however, this is only a starting point. For effective and healthy meal planning we suggest consulting a nutritionist and/or doctor that specializes in overeating problems.

Biological Plan

1. My healthy meal plan, including portion control, consists of the following: _____

   _____

   _____

2. Old eating patterns I plan to avoid and replace with healthy patterns are: _____

   _____

   _____

3. My healthy meal schedule is: _____

_____

_____

Psychological Plan

PART ONE: Three thinking patterns that triggered overeating in the past and challenging self-talk:

Addictive Thinking Pattern	Challenging Self-Talk
1.	1a.
2.	2a..
3.	3a.

PART TWO: Three emotions that triggered overeating in the past and healthy feeling management strategies:

Triggering Emotions	Managment Strategies
1.	1a.
2.	2a..
3.	3a.

PART THREE: Three behaviors that triggered or worsened overeating in the past and healthy changes:

Triggering Behaviors	Managment Strategies
1.	1a.
2.	2a..
3.	3a.

Social Plan

Three social/intimate situations that have been problematic in the past and healthy coping strategies:

Social/Intimate Triggers	Managment Strategies
1.	1a.
2.	2a..
3.	3a.

Spiritual Plan

Three spiritual triggers that have been problematic in the past and healthy coping strategies:

Spiritual Triggers	Managment Strategies
1.	1a.
2.	2a..
3.	3a.

What is the most important thing you learned as a result of completing this exercise?

_____

_____

What are you willing to do differently as a result of what you learned in this exercise?

_____

_____

This exercise stops here.

Exercise 2: Creating Your Personalized Definition of Abstinence

Part 1: What Is Abstinence?

The goal of this exercise is to help you clearly define your bottom line for abstinence (sobriety) from compulsive or addictive eating, whether your behaviors include overeating, skipping meals, grazing, etc. While your Healthy Living Plan is a "progress, not perfection" plan, you can follow your abstinent definition 100 percent of the time, just as the alcoholic abstains from drinking alcohol 100 percent of the time (Jackson, B. 2000. *Dieting, a Dry Drunk.* Universal Publishers).

When you arrest your compulsive eating patterns, you will find that the rest of your Healthy Living Plan will be much easier to follow and enjoy. This process might seem frightening at first. Please remember that you're not alone, and this step in your recovery will set you free!

Your final definition should be clear and concise and only relate to your personal eating patterns. Examples might look like this: "I eat three planned and moderate meals daily and nothing in between" or "I eat five moderate meals daily and don't skip any meals."

Part 2: Developing Your Personalized Definition

Let's take a look at the behaviors that have been most problematic for you and plan the most simple and clear definition of abstinence possible:

1. List below the five (5) most problematic eating patterns you experience (include night-time eating, grazing, skipping a particular meal, purging calories through exercise, etc.):
   - _____
   - _____
   - _____
   - _____
   - _____

2. What number of meals per day does your lifestyle support and why? Our society is primarily set up for three meals daily, but that is variable for some of us. What makes sense for you?

   _____

   _____

   _____

3. As a result of the answers from the questions above, create your definition of abstinence now:

   _____

   _____

   _____

4. Look at your definition: Is it simple? Is it something you can follow 100 percent of the time? Does it feel like a diet when you read it? Please explain: _____

_____

_____

_____

Part 3: Finalizing Your Personalized Definition of Abstinence

Read your definition above. If it feels like a diet plan you're creating to try to lose weight, go back and start over. Weight loss is not your goal! Recovery is. With a moderate and balanced plan of eating, you will naturally experience both physical and emotional relief.

We suggest that you lovingly create this definition for yourself. If you find yourself struggling, pretend that you are doing this for a dear friend who is recovering from a long life-threatening illness and desperately needs your help.

My final personalized definition for abstinence is:

_____

_____

_____

**Go to the next page and complete
Your Definition of Abstinence Summary.**

Part 4: Your Definition of Abstinence Summary

INSTRUCTIONS: Before your next group or individual session, take a few minutes to complete the following items, and be prepared to share (not read) your reactions to the previous exercise.

1. As I was completing the exercise, I was thinking: _____

    _____

    _____

    _____

2. As I was completing the exercise, I was feeling: _____

    _____

    _____

    _____

3. The level or risk of an eating addiction that I rated myself at was _____. I rated myself that way because: _____

    _____

    _____

    _____

4. The most important thing I learned as a result of completing this exercise was: _____

    _____

    _____

    _____

5. What I plan to do differently as a result of completing this exercise is:

    _____

    _____

    _____

This exercise stops here.

Exercise 3: Eating Addiction Problem Checklist

INSTRUCTIONS: Almost everyone overeats sometimes, but most people stop when they become uncomfortable. Some can't/don't stop even in the face of consequences. When people start to use eating addictively/compulsively, they begin to have problems. These problems are often described as the *symptoms* of an eating addiction/compulsion. Answer each question below as honestly as you can. You may notice some of the questions will make you feel uncomfortable. As a matter of fact, you may notice you have an urge to lie about (rationalize or minimize) your answers. If this happens, it means you have an urge to deny the problems related to your compulsive eating. If this is the case, it may be helpful to talk to a counselor or sponsor about the questions that cause an urge to minimize, rationalize, or deny an issue around eating. These feelings are information and clues about your personal relationship to eating. Use a checkmark to note the questions that make you feel uncomfortable, and talk about them with your sponsor or counselor.

The goal of having you answer these questions is to give you a chance to think about some of the problems you may have experienced with eating. To make these questions helpful for you, take the time to think and talk about your answers. Also notice the feelings that each question provokes. Some of these questions may raise concerns in your own mind or may make you start arguing with yourself. ***These are important questions to discuss with someone else. If you are currently in recovery or abstinent, please think back and answer the following questions as you would when your eating addiction was at its worst.***

❑ Yes ❑ No   1. Do you find yourself eating, although you are not really hungry?

❑ Yes ❑ No   2. Do you ever hide how much you eat from others?

❑ Yes ❑ No   3. Have you ever eaten to cope with feelings or to manage stress?

❑ Yes ❑ No   4. Have you had a persistent desire or made unsuccessful efforts to cut down or control your eating patterns?

❑ Yes ❑ No   5. Do you often eat more, or differently, than you originally intended?

❑ Yes ❑ No   6. Have you been told you had to lose weight because of a medical problem and been unable to do so?

❑ Yes ❑ No   7. If you were told you had to stop your compulsive/addictive eating use because of a medical problem, would it be difficult for you to stop?

❑ Yes❑ No   8. Have friends/family expressed concern or confronted you about your overeating and/or weight issues?

❑ Yes ❑ No   9. Have you ever continued eating compulsively/addictively even though you knew it was causing problems or making your problems worse?

❑ Yes ❑ No   10. Do you ever use nonprescribed drugs to control your appetite or weight? (These might include medicines like diet pills, sleep aids, caffeine, stay-awake pills, herbal supplements, or cigarette smoking, etc.)

❑ Yes ❑ No   11. Do you have a history of using prescription drugs to lose weight?

❑ Yes ❑ No   12. Do you ever feel self-conscious, guilty, or ashamed when eating—even *normal* eating?

❑ Yes ❑ No   13. Do you spend a great deal of your time thinking about what you are going to eat, where to get it, and then feeling badly after eating it?

❑ Yes ❑ No 14. Have you lost your enthusiasm for living because of your eating or weight?

❑ Yes ❑ No 15. Do you eat to avoid or delay your human feelings: having normal body functions, needing sleep, feeling sexual, finishing a project, having fun, etc.?

❑ Yes ❑ No 16. Have you ever felt guilty or ashamed around your eating issues, e.g., binge eating, sneaking food, stealing food, retrieving food that has been thrown away, eating off other people's plates, out of garbage cans?

❑ Yes ❑ No 17. Have you experienced depression or even thoughts of suicide because of your overeating or the resulting physical, emotional, or weight problems?

❑ Yes ❑ No 18. Have you ever skipped breakfast because you were so full from the night before?

❑ Yes ❑ No 19. Do you ever go without eating all day just to find yourself bingeing throughout the evening/night?

❑ Yes ❑ No 20. Have you ever attended self-help meetings or counseling to deal with eating or weight problems?

❑ Yes ❑ No 21. Have you ever been too sick to go to work as a result of bingeing? (This includes eating withdrawal-like symptoms, such as exhaustion; being bloated; feeling hungover, irritable, overactive, or unable to concentrate.)

❑ Yes ❑ No 22. Have you ever withheld information from your doctor about another doctor's (or other healthcare provider's) warnings regarding your weight or related health issues?

❑ Yes ❑ No 23. Do you ever eat just to numb out or feel high?

❑ Yes ❑ No 24. Have you ever felt sick, anxious, hypersensitive, or headachy (or experienced other *eating withdrawal* symptoms) when you suddenly stopped overeating or stopped eating certain foods?

❑ Yes ❑ No 25. Have you ever been in a hospital as a (direct or indirect) result of your eating addiction? For example, high cholesterol; diabetes; obesity; back, knee, or foot problems; heart attack; etc.

❑ Yes ❑ No 26. Have you felt shame and/or been angry with your spouse, family members, or close friends because they commented on your eating or weight?

❑ Yes ❑ No 27. Have you ever failed to finish home or work commitments because you were bingeing on food or were in withdrawal?

❑ Yes ❑ No 28. Have you ever let other people down (either those close to you or at work) or just couldn't be bothered because you were binge eating or hungover?

❑ Yes ❑ No 29. Do you believe that *only* eating can comfort you and get you through difficult times?

❑ Yes ❑ No 30. Does your pattern of eating and its negative consequences ever affect your sex/love life or make you too ashamed to participate or be really present?

Go to the next page for Interpreting the
Eating Addiction Problem Checklist.

Part 1: Interpreting the Eating Addiction Problem Checklist

Please add up the number of yes answers: _____

Directions: Please check the box of the statement below that most applies to your score on the above questions.

❑ If you answered no to all of the above, you probably do not have an eating addiction.

❑ If you answered yes to three to five of the above, you may have an eating addiction.

❑ If you answered yes to six to eight of the above, you probably do have an eating addiction.

❑ If you answered yes to nine to twelve of the above, you definitely have an eating addiction.

❑ If you answered yes to thirteen or more of the above, you have a serious eating addiction.

Do you agree with the results of the interpretation of the Eating Addiction Checklist?

❑ Yes ❑ No ❑ Unsure   Please explain: _____

_____

_____

_____

Go to the next page and complete the Checklist Summary.

Part 2: Eating Addiction Problem Checklist Summary

INSTRUCTIONS: Before your next group or individual session, take a few minutes to complete the following items and be prepared to share (not read) your reactions to the previous exercise.

1. As I was completing the exercise I was thinking: _____

    _____

    _____

    _____

2. As I was completing the exercise I was feeling: _____

    _____

    _____

    _____

3. The level or risk of an eating addiction that I rated myself at was _____ . I rated myself that way because: _____

    _____

    _____

    _____

4. The most important thing I learned as a result of completing this exercise was:

    _____

    _____

    _____

5. What I plan to do differently as a result of completing this exercise is:

    _____

    _____

    _____

This exercise stops here.

27

Exercise 4: Decision Making

Part 1: What You Wanted

Please answer each of the following questions as fully and honestly as you can.

1. What are the three most important things you wanted eating to do for you?

   A._____

   B._____

   C._____

2. Could you have done these things for yourself without eating compulsively/addictively?

   ❑   Yes   ❑   No   ❑   Unsure   Please explain: _____

   _____

   _____

   _____

3. What are the three most important things you wanted eating to help you cope with or escape from?

   A._____

   B._____

   C._____

4. Can you cope with or escape from these things without eating compulsively/addictively?

   ❑   Yes   ❑   No   ❑   Unsure   Please explain: _____

   _____

   _____

   _____

5. Looking back on it now, do you think that eating did for you what you wanted it to do?

   ❑   Yes   ❑   No   ❑   Unsure   Please explain: _____

   _____

   _____

Go to Part 2 and complete the exercise—What You Learned.

Part 2: What You Learned

1. Please list below the three most important things you have learned as a result of completing this exercise.

    A._____

    _____

    B._____

    _____

    C._____

    _____

2. What do you plan to do differently as a result of completing this exercise?

    _____

    _____

    _____

> **Go to Part 3 and complete the exercise—The Decision to
> Stop Using Eating as a Coping Tool.**

Part 3: The Decision to Stop Using Eating as a Coping Tool

When you are confronted with a decision to make a significant lifestyle change, it is very important to carefully weigh the pros and cons (i.e., benefits and disadvantages) of making that transition. It is easy for many people who have been eating compulsively/addictively to see the disadvantages or negative consequences of that behavior (e.g., obesity, heart problems, joint problems). But it is more difficult for them to admit to the benefits of eating addictively.

Some people use eating to cope with uncomfortable emotions or to deal with the consequences of having poor social skills and lack of friendships. Others use eating to avoid intimacy by making food their best friend. There must be some benefits to your eating compulsively/addictively or you wouldn't have started using eating to cope instead of for fuel. These benefits are sometimes called *secondary gains*. Before you complete the following worksheet below, you might find it helpful to go back and review *Exercise 1: Creating Your Healthy Living Plan* and look at how you used eating as a coping tool in the biopsychosocialspiritual areas. With this in mind, please complete the following worksheet.

The Benefits and Disadvantages of Eating Compulsively/Addictively

1. **Benefits**—List the main things that were better or easier for you because you ate compulsively.	2. **Disadvantages:**—List the main things that were worse for you or problems that you had because you ate compulsively.

3. Looking back on it, do you think that the benefits you expected from eating compulsively/addictively were worth the pain and problems you experienced?

❑ Yes ❑ No ❑ Unsure Please explain: _____

_____

_____

> **Go to the next page and complete the
> Decision Making Summary.**

30

Part 4: Decision Making Summary

INSTRUCTIONS: Before your next group or individual session take a few minutes to complete the following items and be prepared to share (not read) your reactions to the previous exercise.

1. As I was completing the exercises, I was thinking:

    _____

    _____

    _____

2. As I was completing the exercises, I was feeling:

    _____

    _____

    _____

3. What were the major benefits and disadvantages that you noted?

    _____

    _____

    _____

4. The most important thing I learned as a result of completing this exercise was:

    _____

    _____

    _____

5. What I plan to do differently as a result of completing this exercise is:

    _____

    _____

    _____

This exercise stops here.

Exercise 5: Intervention Planning

Part 1: Craving Intervention Planning

When you have made a decision to take action, become abstinent, and follow a Healthy Living Plan, there is a strong possibility you may experience intense urges or cravings to once again use eating to cope with stress or for comfort. This doesn't mean you are weak or don't have a commitment to follow your healthy living contract. It is normal for people who quit using eating compulsively/addictively to have thoughts and even strong cravings to fall back into old ways.

There are some action steps you can take to avoid relapsing into old behaviors by creating an effective craving management plan. Below are nine generic examples of steps you can take to avoid giving in to your cravings. As you read each of the interventions below, rate your ability to implement each one on a scale of 1 to 10, with 1 meaning "I would not be able to do that" and 10 meaning "I could definitely do that."

1. **Recognize and Accept:** Recognize the craving and accept it as a normal part of recovery. Remind yourself that just because you're having a craving does not mean there is something wrong with you. It is normal to have cravings. _____

2. **Decide Not to Act on the Craving:** Tell yourself the following: "No matter what happens, I'm not going to act on this craving. Instead I'll call someone. Cravings go away whether I give in to them or not. I have proven this before and I can do what it takes to shut this down." _____

3. **Change the Physical Setting:** Change your physical and/or social location—**GET OUT OF THERE!** Sometimes something as simple as changing chairs makes a big difference. Don't be around people who apply negative peer pressure. Hang with positive recovery-prone people. _____

4. **Meditation and Relaxation:** Learn simple relaxation and/or meditation techniques (your counselor can help you with this). Sometimes just taking a few deep breaths can also make a big difference. Some people report great benefit from meditation and/or relaxation cassettes—check them out! Remember, contempt before investigation equals ignorance. _____

5. **Negative Consequences:** Remind yourself of the negative things that will probably happen if you give into your craving and start to eat compulsively/addictively again; try to be mindful of these things before you have any cravings. Remember all the pain and problems you have experienced and the money you have spent as a result of giving in to cravings before. _____

6. **Benefits of Not Eating Compulsively/Addictively:** Remind yourself of all the good things that can happen if you continue to follow your Healthy Living Plan—your personal definition of abstinence. List some of the things that you can now accomplish because you are abstinent that would have been difficult if not impossible to do while eating compulsively/addictively. _____

7. **Exercise:** Have a regular daily pattern of exercise developed, and practice it on an ongoing basis. When you have a craving, begin using one of your exercise activities. _____

8. **Eat Healthy:** Creating your abstinence plan with the help of a certified nutritionist or doctor will be very helpful. Learn how to fuel your body in a healthy way, and avoid your trigger foods as much as possible—especially when having cravings. _____

9. **Mastery Imagery:** Close your eyes and imagine yourself being successful and powerful when you decide not to give in to your cravings. Imagine all the positive benefits you will experience and how good you will feel about yourself for not giving in to the cravings. _____

10. **My Personal Plan:** Try to imagine yourself in a situation where you would begin to experience strong urges or cravings to use eating compulsively/addictively. Then using the above steps as a starting point, please list your step-by-step action plan in the space below. You should have at least four or five solid steps in your plan. Here, more *is* better.

_____

_____

_____

_____

_____

_____

_____

_____

**Go to the next page and learn about
Relapse Intervention Planning.**

Part 2: Relapse Intervention Planning

Relapse Intervention Plan: One of the goals of completing this workbook is to prepare you to quickly stop your use of eating as a coping tool and/or resume working an effective recovery program. This process is called developing a relapse intervention plan. *It is unrealistic to expect you will not experience slips/relapse when dealing with your recovery.*

Factors that stop relapse quickly: Your response to relapse will be determined in large part by the following five factors: (1) what you were told will happen if you start to use eating again as a coping tool or start mismanaging your recovery program; (2) what you can do to stop eating compulsively/addictively and/or get back to using an effective recovery program if relapse occurs; (3) the approach of other people who deal with you after the relapse has occurred; (4) what you say to yourself when you're not "perfect," and (5) knowing what your personal definition of abstinence is, which you developed in *Exercise 2*, so you can get back into full compliance.

Guidelines that stop relapse quickly should it occur: It's a mistaken belief that if you have one compulsive/addictive eating episode, you will lose control and not be able to stop until you hit bottom. There are two reasons not to believe this: First, it's not true. Many recovering people have short-term and low-consequence slips/relapses and get immediately back into full compliance with their definition of abstinence and full recovery before serious damage occurs. Second, this negative approach programs you for a long-term catastrophic relapse episode and increased shame, which makes it even more difficult to ask for help. If you do start eating compulsively/addictively, the misleading voice may pop into your head saying, "If you take one bite of the *wrong* food, you will lose control and not be able to stop until you hit bottom." You may then feel hopeless and/or say to yourself, "Well, I might as well keep going until I hit bottom." *This does not mean it's perfectly fine to "slip"* whenever the mood strikes or as long as your life doesn't fall apart. You still have to be vigilant. This is a high-risk situation. Fortunately, if you do start to use eating as a coping tool, you will hit moments of sanity where you can choose to get help and stop the relapse. At these moments it is important to *act immediately*. If you wait, the urge to use again will come back and the opportunity will be lost. If you do start deviating from your Healthy Living Plan or start to use eating to cope and hit a moment of sanity where you want to stop, the six most effective things for you to do follow:

1. Read your prepared relapse intervention plan, which should always be readily accessible. (You should also give copies to your appropriate significant others so they will be more able to help.)

2. Do not keep a slip/relapse a secret. Secrets and shame support relapse, not recovery.

3. Immediately call for help and get into a recovery supportive situation.

4. Call a counselor or sponsor, go to a treatment program, or get to a support group meeting.

5. In addition to this help, immediately stop eating compulsively/addictively and get out of the situation that supports compulsive/addictive eating.

6. *Please do not try to handle your recovery process alone. If that were possible, you would not need this workbook.*

**Go to the next page and complete
The Relapse Intervention Plan.**

34

The Relapse Intervention Plan: In its simplest form, developing a relapse intervention plan consists of answering the following three questions and creating a specific written plan in response to each question. This is a plan that is created, written, and distributed while you are in recovery following your Healthy Living Plan and thinking clearly.

1. What is your counselor, doctor, and/or sponsor supposed to do if you relapse, stop coming to sessions, or fail to honor your abstinence commitment and Healthy Living Contract? What would help the most?

    _____

    _____

    _____

2. What are you going to do to get back in recovery if you start eating to cope or deviate from your abstinence commitment and Healthy Living Plan—so that you can stop the slip/relapse quickly?

    _____

    _____

3. Who are three significant others who have an investment in your recovery, and what are they supposed to do if relapse occurs? Make sure you have their day and night phone numbers accessible, and give them a copy of this plan.

    A. Name of Significant Other #1: _____ Phone: _____

    What are they supposed to do? What would help the most?

    _____

    _____

    B. Name of Significant Other #2: _____ Phone: _____

    What are they supposed to do? What would help the most?

    _____

    _____

    C. Name of Significant Other #3: _____ Phone: _____

    What are they supposed to do? What would help the most?

    _____

    _____

**Go to the next page and complete
The Intervention Plan Summary.**

Part 3: The Intervention Plan Summary

INSTRUCTIONS: Before your next group or individual session, take a few minutes to complete the following items and be prepared to share (not read) your reactions to the previous exercise.

1. As I was completing the exercises, I was thinking: _____

    _____

    _____

    _____

2. As I was completing the exercises, I was feeling: _____

    _____

    _____

    _____

3. What were the most important interventions you developed? _____

    _____

    _____

    _____

4. The most important thing I learned as a result of completing this exercise was:

    _____

    _____

    _____

5. What I plan to do differently as a result of completing this exercise is: _____

    _____

    _____

    _____

This exercise stops here.

Exercise 6: The Healthy Living Contract

Part 1: Presenting Problems

1. **Presenting problems:** What are the presenting problems that caused you to seek help at this time? (Why did you seek help now? Why not yesterday or next week? What would have happened if you didn't seek help now? What problems or negative consequences can this workbook help you to avoid or resolve?)

   _____

   _____

   _____

   _____

2. **Relationship to compulsive/addictive eating:** How is each presenting problem related to your compulsive/addictive eating (i.e., using eating as a coping tool) and/or to an ineffective lifestyle?
   How is this problem related to your compulsive/addictive eating? Did eating compulsively/ addictively cause you to have this problem? (Would you have this problem if you never ate compulsively/addictively or used eating as a coping tool?) Did compulsive/ addictive eating make this problem worse than it would have been if you hadn't been using it that way? Or did eating compulsively/addictively lead you to mistakenly believe that it helped you to cope with the problem?

   _____

   _____

   _____

   _____

3. **Consequences of not stopping:** What additional problems could you experience if you keep eating compulsively/addictively as a coping tool despite these problems? (What are the benefits? What are the disadvantages? What is the best thing that could happen? What is the worst? What is the most probable thing that will happen?)

   _____

   _____

   _____

   _____

4. **Asking for a commitment toward health (The Healthy Eating Commitment):** Are you willing to make a commitment to use an eating plan that is healthy for you (not as a coping tool) and adhere to your definition of abstinence for *<name the specific period of time:* _____>? (This should be done with the assistance of your doctor, counselor, sponsor, or other support person.)

   ❑ Yes   ❑ No   ❑ Unsure   Please explain: _____

   _____

   _____

   _____

5. **Immediate high-risk situations:** Are you facing any situations in the near future that could cause you to want to eat compulsively/addictively despite your commitment not to?

   ❑ Yes   ❑ No   ❑ Unsure   Please explain: _____

   _____

   _____

   _____

6. **Your commitment:** Are you willing to make an agreement to complete the following exercises in order to learn how to identify and manage those high-risk situations without eating compulsively/addictively or using it as a coping tool?

   ❑ Yes   ❑ No   ❑ Unsure   Please explain: _____

   _____

   _____

   _____

**Go to the next page and complete the
Presenting Problem Summary.**

Part 2: Presenting Problem Summary

INSTRUCTIONS: Before your next group or individual session, take a few minutes to complete the following report form, and be prepared to share (not read) your reactions to the previous exercise.

My Presenting Problems	How Does My Compulsive/Addictive Eating Relate to This Problem?	Consequences if I Keep Eating in This Way

Go to the next page for
Competing the Healthy Living Contract.

Part 3: Completing the Healthy Living Contract

I, _____, do hereby agree to the following terms and conditions of treatment.

1. **Healthy Living Plan:** I agree to my Healthy Living Plan developed in a previous exercise as long as I am receiving service/help from _____.

2. **Adhering to Abstinence:** I agree to completely adhere to my own personal definition of abstinence that I developed in *Exercise 2* of this workbook.

3. **High-Risk Situations:** I agree to immediately tell my counselor, sponsor, or other appropriate support person about any problems or situations that may develop that could cause me to start eating compulsively/addictively or to deviate from my definition of abstinence despite my commitment.

4. **Cravings or Urges to Eat Compulsively/Addictively:** I agree to immediately discuss any cravings or urges to eat compulsively/addictively with my counselor, sponsor, or appropriate support person.

5. **Desire to Stop Treatment:** I agree to immediately discuss any thoughts or feelings I may have about wanting to stop treatment sessions or stop participating in other recovery activities, such as self-help groups.

6. **Self-Reporting of Relapse:** I agree that if I do start eating compulsively/addictively or deviating from my personal definition of abstinence, I will immediately report it to my counselor, sponsor, or appropriate support person. After reporting my relapse the following will happen: (1) My current treatment plan (or recovery plan) will be immediately suspended. (2) I will be asked to complete a new evaluation to determine what treatment (or recovery plan) is necessary to stop the relapse. (3) I will be given a treatment or recovery recommendation (that may include referral for a more intensive or extended outpatient program). (4) If I refuse the recommendation, I may be terminated from treatment, or, if this is with a sponsor, they may choose to stop working with me.

7. **Prescribed Medications:** I will consult with treatment program staff or my healthcare provider team member regarding the use of any medications prescribed to me by any other healthcare provider. I will follow the recommendations of the assigned medical staff of the treatment program or my healthcare team member regarding the use of any and all mood-altering or diet medication.

8. I also agree to the following interventions developed in my Healthy Living Plan and Craving Plan:

_____

_____

_____

_____

_____

_____

_____

_____

_____

_____

_____   _____   _____   _____
Signature of Client   Date   Signature of Witness   Date

This "Healthy Living" contract was adapted from the abstinence contract developed and field tested by Terence T. Gorski and CENAPS® Trainer/Consultant, Tim Dworniczek, for chemical dependency treatment.

Go to the next page and complete
The Healthy Living Contract Summary.

Part 4: The Healthy Living Contract Summary

INSTRUCTIONS: Before your next group or individual session, take a few minutes to complete the following items, and be prepared to share (not read) your reactions to the previous exercise.

1. As I was completing the exercises, I was thinking: _____

   _____

   _____

   _____

2. As I was completing the exercises, I was feeling: _____

   _____

   _____

   _____

3. What were the major presenting problems you listed? _____

   _____

   _____

   _____

4. The most important thing I learned as a result of completing this exercise was: _____

   _____

   _____

   _____

5. What I plan to do differently as a result of completing this exercise is: _____

   _____

   _____

   _____

This exercise stops here.

Exercise 7: High-Risk Situations

Part 1: Identifying High-Risk Situations

A high-risk situation is any experience that can activate the urge to deviate from your personal definition of abstinence or use eating as a coping tool instead of fuel, despite your commitment not to. It could be a situation that makes you want to stop using your effective recovery program despite your promises to yourself. Defining the concept of a high-risk situation can be tricky. Some situations activate self-defeating urges for *some* people, but not for others. The same situation can activate the urges at some *times*, but not others. So how do you describe what a high-risk situation is? This exercise is designed to help you identify a high-risk situation you will be facing in the near future and personalize it. You will do this by completing the following items.

1. **Identify your immediate high-risk situation.** Think ahead over the next two to four weeks and identify a situation that could make you want to deviate from your personal definition of abstinence or use eating as a coping tool (compulsively/addictively) instead of for fuel, despite your commitment not to. Write a short sentence that describes this situation. What is the situation?

   _____

   _____

2. **How does this situation increase your risk of eating compulsively/addictively?** Write a sentence or short paragraph that describes how this situation will make you want to deviate from your personal definition of abstinence or to eat compulsively/addictively despite your commitment.

   _____

   _____

3. **Write a personal title.** Write a personal title for that situation. (A title is a word or short phrase that identifies the situation.) "Getting Complacent" and "Shame Spiral" are sample titles for the example description in #4.

   Personal Title: _____

4. **Write a personal description.** Write a sentence that describes your high-risk situation. Use this format: *I know that I am in a high-risk situation when **<I do something>** that causes **<pain and problems>** and I want to eat to manage the pain or to solve the problems. (Example: I know that I am in a high-risk situation when **<I stop exercising daily>** and that causes **<my weight to increase>** so I feel ashamed and want to eat to make me feel better.)*

   _____

   _____

   _____

5. **Risk of mismanaging the high-risk situation:** How high a risk is it for you to deviate from your personal definition of abstinence, to eat compulsively/addictively, or use other self-defeating behaviors to manage this situation? (Please circle the number of your choice on the following scale.)

0–3 = no or low risk, 4–6 = moderate risk (50/50 chance), 7–10 = high to very high risk

0 --------- 1 --------- 2 --------- 3 --------- 4 --------- 5 --------- 6 --------- 7 --------- 8 --------- 9 --------- 10

6. Why do you rate your risk at this level? Please explain: _____

_____

_____

_____

**Please go to the next page to read
The Eating Addiction High-Risk Situation List.**

Part 2: The Eating Addiction High-Risk Situation List

An eating addiction is eating food to help us cope with life situations, instead of eating only for fueling our bodies. A high-risk situation is something that happens that makes us want to eat to cope—even after making a commitment not to—causing a *relapse* to our addiction. Or it's a situation that makes us want to stop using our Healthy Living Plan (recovery program) and return to our old ways of coping that could also include eating compulsively/addictively. We don't get into high-risk situations by accident. We may feel drawn to these situations. On some level we surrender our power and start believing we are a victim again, telling ourselves, "This is too hard." You could say we start going SOUR (Setting Ourselves Up to Relapse). Once we're in the situation, we mistakenly believe that we don't know what to do, or we respond with our old automatic and unconscious habits. We convince ourselves that it's really not our fault, we didn't plan it, it just happened, and there's nothing we can do about it anyway. What follows are some high-risk situations that others have discovered were problems for them. ***If you are currently stable with your Healthy Living Plan, please rate the high-risk situations as you would in the past or as you would if you find yourself in a relapse mode in the future.***

Instructions:

*As you read each of the high-risk situations (HRS), **please rate each on a scale of 0 to 10**—with 0 meaning this has not, does not, and probably will not apply to me and 10 meaning that it has been, is, or could be a serious problem for me. Keep in mind that you may have an urge to minimize or rationalize these situations, or even feel upset by what you read. If this happens to you, please be sure to share this reaction with someone you trust.*

❑   1.   **We don't feel connected:** We may be so self-conscious, because of our weight or eating obsession, that we have difficulty connecting with others. When we are obsessed with eating, it may be difficult to focus on anything or anyone else.

❑   2.   **We seek temporary fixes:** We want to control our eating and our weight to prepare us for some special event or circumstance (e.g., a reunion, a wedding, a first date). We may often do crash diets or fasts to achieve some of those short-term goals. We mistakenly believe that if we can achieve our goal weight by controlling our eating, then we really don't have a problem—we just needed the motivation.

❑   3.   **We don't make the connection:** We don't see the relationship between our eating patterns and the problems that we're experiencing. We convince ourselves that we need to continue to eat the way we want to despite our problems. We admit to ourselves that we've got some serious problems—that's why we eat the way we do, to help us cope with them.

❑   4.   **We tend to isolate:** Perhaps we are shy and uncomfortable around others, so we make food our friend and we have a relationship with the way we eat it. Or maybe when we have a craving to eat, we push people away so we can be left in peace to eat what we want, the way we want, how much we want, and when we want.

❑   5.   **We have nostalgic memories about eating:** We start remembering how comforting it was to eat all we wanted or to eat certain foods and not worry about the consequences (e.g., putting on weight, how badly we may hate ourselves, how sick and bloated we may feel).

❑   6.   **We deny we have a problem:** We tell ourselves that we're in control of our eating; it doesn't control us. We can stop any time we want to—but it doesn't dawn on us

45

that we never want to. Besides, we're not engaging in our old coping styles right now and that proves we're in control.

❑ 7. **We *cannot* imagine living without our comfort foods:** We start thinking about how hard it is to stay away from the eating behaviors and food that used to comfort us. We convince ourselves that it is unbearable to have to live without our old ways of coping. This new way of living is too hard and uncomfortable; besides, we'll never be able to really enjoy life without eating what we want, when we want it.

❑ 8. **We fool ourselves:** We mistakenly believe that eating can distract us and help us cope with painful situations. We convince ourselves that we won't lose control. We'll be responsible and eat just a little. Besides, it will just be this one time. We'll only use the old way of eating for a short period of time until the pressure is off. Then we'll stop and get back to our recovery/abstinence and our Healthy Living Plan.

❑ 9. **We make our problems worse:** Sometimes we have legitimate problems that need to be dealt with, but we engage in self-defeating behaviors that make them worse instead of better. We indulge in feelings of self-pity and try to avoid the problem, but we realize it doesn't really work. Instead of solving our problems (or facing our feelings), we spiral downward and eventually start to eat compulsively/addictively again.

❑ 10. **We overcommit:** Sometimes we take on more than we can handle and start missing deadlines and letting other people down. Instead of talking openly about the problem, we go underground, put things off, blame others, and try to cover our tracks. When we get caught, we get defensive and try to talk our way out of it; we end up feeling really bad about ourselves. To escape, we start eating compulsively/addictively because that seems to be our best or only way out.

❑ 11. **We get frustrated:** Sometimes we get frustrated because we want to eat something that others have told us we shouldn't have, or we made a promise not to. When this happens, we feel deprived because we should be able to have it, just this once. Besides, we have the right to change our mind, and it's none of their business anyway.

❑ 12. **We deserve a treat:** There are times when we start to convince ourselves that deviating from our Healthy Living Plan just a little would be all right. Besides, we really do deserve something for all our hard work. We've been good for so long; we're entitled to it. Nobody has the right to tell us we can't reward ourselves.

❑ 13. **We argue and fight:** Sometimes when we visit our friends, other family members, or our parents, we end up getting into arguments or conflicts. We leave believing that no one really cares about us or understands us. We then have an urge to use eating to soothe ourselves.

❑ 14. **We put ourselves in high-risk situations:** For example, being around free food, potlucks, all-you-can-eat promotions, and buying bulk—because we get more for our money—places us in situations of high risk.

❑ 15. **We want to change how we feel:** We might get into situations that stress us out or make us feel angry, tired, or bored. We mistakenly believe that we need to eat to either calm us down or to pick us up. We forget there is a better, healthier way, and we don't implement our Healthy Living Plan.

□ 16. **We see other people enjoying themselves:** We might be in a social situation where people are overeating and we want to join in. We suddenly notice that everyone else is indulging and having a really good time. We don't want to eat this way, but everyone else is and we feel pressured to do it as well. But more than that, we feel deprived. We remember how good it felt to eat what we wanted and ask ourselves, "Why not?" Besides everyone else is overeating, so no one will notice we're doing it.

□ 17. **We face a loss:** A family member or friend might die. We have to go to the funeral and attend the social functions that surround it where we see people eating and using alcohol or other drugs to cope with their pain. There are comfort foods (e.g., chocolate, pastries, ice cream) being passed around to anyone who wants them. We remember how eating and other coping behaviors helped us feel better in the past. Then we go home, alone, to deal with our pain and loss. We want to feel better, but we don't know how to do it without eating compulsively/addictively.

□ 18. **We remember bad experiences:** We might get into situations that remind us of a painful past situation—such as an early childhood trauma, a major failure or loss, a personal trauma or tragedy—and we are overwhelmed with feelings. We hurt and don't know how to deal with the pain or if we even want to. We have an urge to eat so we don't have to feel any of it.

□ 19. **We feel trapped:** A situation may come up that backs us into a corner, and we start feeling trapped because we don't know how to handle it. We don't want to admit we can't handle situations, so we begin isolating and feel cutoff from others. It seems like there is no way to fit in or get connected. To avoid situations like this, we might start spending more time alone. And when we're by ourselves, we might start to feel lonely and have urges to eat.

□ 20. **We judge ourselves and feel shame:** When we go out shopping, we try to avoid looking in the mirror. But sometimes we are confronted with what we believe is an unappealing reflection of ourselves. Sometimes we may not be able to find anything we believe looks good on us. We start thinking that something's wrong with us, because we don't match the image of what the fashion industry says an attractive man/woman should look like. We feel flawed and defective. Our self-perception becomes distorted and we see ourselves larger or smaller than we really are.

□ 21. **We fear holidays or other eating-oriented occasions:** We know that everyone around us will be overindulging, and we may be confronted with temptations that we ordinarily avoid. Everywhere we go we are bombarded with sights, sounds, and smells that fuel our addictive thinking process. We find ourselves longing to be a normal eater who can occasionally indulge and then stop. We know that's not possible and we begin to feel angry. We isolate and then feel sorry for ourselves about being alone.

□ 22. **We fail to eat at appropriate times:** Despite all that we know about eating at regular intervals, we sometimes skip meals. Then we justify a larger lunch and/or night bingeing or grazing. We mistakenly believe it's OK to skip a meal (especially breakfast), then we give ourselves permission to eat more than we should at a later time (setting up our next binge).

□ 23. **We eat in weird places:** We want to appear to be normal eaters in the presence of other people. Sometimes we hide how much or how often we eat by eating the extra food in less public places (e.g., in our car, before/after going out to dinner, before going to bed, before/after socializing). We may also hide how we eat—gobbling, bingeing, digging food out of the trash, eating frozen foods before thawing, etc.

❑ 24. **We consider food our friend or lover:** The process of eating is the relationship we have with food—our only safe companionship. Because it seems to need nothing back, we mistakenly believe we are satisfied, physically and emotionally. It may feel like a physical hug.

❑ 25. **We must clean our plate or else:** We grew up as members of the clean-plate club and feel guilty any time we leave food on a plate, because of the messages we received as children about wasting food. Some of us may have even been punished for not eating every bite.

❑ 26. **We struggle with transitions, even the good ones:** Sometimes we find ourselves feeling hungry when we start or leave a job, begin or end a relationship, achieve or give up on a long-term goal. We may finally achieve our cherished goal, but no matter what transitions are going on in our lives, we feel hungry and forget to ask ourselves what we're really hungry for.

❑ 27. **We are living with chronic pain or illness:** We might be injured, ill, or experience a chronic pain condition that radically impacts our quality of life. Maybe we can't exercise the way we want or do other things that we used to enjoy. We might even put on weight because we find eating can soothe us. We rationalize this self-destructive pattern of eating, because, after all, we need to have some comfort and relief. We feel guilty and ashamed then use eating to dull the pain.

This Eating Addiction High-Risk Situation (HRS) List was adapted by Dr. Stephen F. Grinstead, Ellen Gruber-Grinstead, and Dr. Shari Stillman-Corbitt from the Food Addiction HRS List developed by Stephen Grinstead, Kay Holmes, and Gabrielle Antolovich, for the original *Food Addiction Workbook* by Stephen Grinstead and Terence T. Gorski, with Kay Holmes and Gabrielle Antolovich.

**Go to the next page and complete the
High-Risk Situation Summary Discussion Questions.**

Part 3: High-Risk Situation Summary Discussion Questions

INSTRUCTIONS: Before your next group or individual session, take a few minutes to complete the following discussion questions, and be prepared to share (not read) your reactions to the previous exercise.

1. What is the high-risk situation you will be facing in the immediate future (during the next two to four weeks) that could cause you to return to your old ways of coping despite your commitment not to? Some people will keep the same situation they identified in Part 1, while others will pick a new situation from something they learned by reading *The Eating Addiction High-Risk Situation List.*

    _____

    _____

2. How did *The Eating Addiction High-Risk Situation List* help you to understand and clarify your immediate high-risk situation? (Or which situation stood out the most for you?)

    _____

    _____

3. Develop a new personal title for your high-risk situation, or maybe modify the one you already chose if it's not quite right. If it still works for you, keep it. Try to find words that are descriptive and easy for you to remember. It should also stir up a feeling or emotion. The title should not be any longer than two or three words. The following are sample titles for the example description in #4 below: "Fooling Myself" or "Failed Again."

    What is a personal title for your high-risk situation?

    _____

4. Develop a *personal description* for the high-risk situation that you selected. The description should start with the words *I know that I'm in a high-risk situation when...* You should use something you learned by reading the high-risk situation list to make the description concrete and specific. Please use the following general format: *(Example: I know that I am in a high-risk situation when <I go to a party> and I don't plan ahead, which leads me < to give into temptation>. Once I start, I tell myself I've blown it, so I might as well just eat what I want.)*

    > *I know that I am in a high-risk situation when* **<I do something or get involved in something regarding a set-up for eating problems>** *that causes* **<pain and problems>** *and I want to use my old coping behaviors to manage the pain and solve the problems.*

    What is a personal description for your high-risk situation?

    _____

    _____

49

5   **Belief in your ability to manage this situation without eating compulsively/addictively:**
How strongly do you believe you will be able to manage this situation without deviating
from your definition of abstinence, eating compulsively/addictively, or disregarding your
Healthy Living Plan?

(Circle the number of your choice below.)

0 = I definitely will **NOT** deviate;   **5** = 50/50 chance of deviating;   **10** = I definitely **WILL** deviate

0 --------- 1 --------- 2 --------- 3 --------- 4 --------- 5 --------- 6 ---------- 7 --------- 8 --------- 9 -------- 10

Why do you rate it this way? _____

_____

_____

6. **Belief in your ability to avoid the situation:** How strongly do you believe you will be
able to avoid getting into this situation?

0 = I definitely will **NOT** avoid it;   **5** = 50/50 chance of avoiding it;   **10** = I definitely WILL avoid it

0 --------- 1 --------- 2 --------- 3 --------- 4 --------- 5 --------- 6 ---------- 7 --------- 8 --------- 9 -------- 10

Why do you rate it this way? _____

_____

_____

7. **Please list at least four interventions** (recovery plans) you can put in place to identify
and manage this and other future high-risk situations that will allow you to continue
following your Healthy Living Plan and make better choices? This will just be a starting
point, because you will develop a more in-depth plan in *Exercise Ten, Recovery Planning*.

What are your four interventions? _____

_____

_____

_____

_____

This exercise stops here.

Exercise 8: Situation Mapping

Part 1: Mapping an Ineffectively Managed Situation

1. Think of a specific time when you experienced this (or a similar) high-risk situation and managed it in a way that caused you to deviate from your definition of abstinence, eat compulsively/addictively, and/or use ineffective recovery planning. Tell the experience as if it were a story with a beginning, middle, and ending. (Start with the phrase: *"The high-risk situation began when..."* Continue step by step. Start describing each step with the words: *"The next thing that happened was..."* End the story with a final statement starting with the words: *"What finally happened was..."*)

   The high-risk situation began when...

   _____

   _____

   _____

   _____

   _____

   _____

   _____

   _____

   _____

   _____

2. What did you want to accomplish by managing this situation the way you did?

   _____

   _____

   _____

3. Did you get what you wanted by managing the situation in this way? If yes, was it worth the cost or negative consequences you experienced?

   ❑ Yes ❑ No ❑ Unsure

   Please explain:

   _____

51

_____

_____

4. On a scale of 1 to 10, what were your stress levels when you managed the situation this way? _____

5. **Doing something different:** Can you think of some things that you could do differently to manage the situation without having to eat compulsively/addictively or deviate from your definition of abstinence?

_____

_____

_____

6. **Avoiding the situation:** What could you have done to responsibly avoid getting into this situation?

_____

_____

_____

If you avoided this situation, how would it have changed the outcome?

_____

_____

_____

7. **Decision point #1:** What could you have done differently near the beginning of the situation to produce a better outcome? (How could you have thought differently? managed your feelings and emotions differently? fought your self-destructive urges differently? acted or behaved differently? treated other people differently?)

_____

_____

_____

If you do these things, how will it change the outcome?

_____

_____

8. **Decision point #2:** What can you do differently near the middle of the situation to produce a better outcome? (How could you have thought differently? managed your feel-

ings and emotions differently? fought your self-destructive urges differently? acted or behaved differently? treated other people differently?)

_____

_____

_____

If you do these things, how will it change the outcome?

_____

_____

9. **Decision point #3:** What can you do differently near the end of the situation to produce a better outcome? (How could you have thought differently? managed your feelings and emotions differently? fought your self-destructive urges differently? acted or behaved differently? treated other people differently?)

_____

_____

_____

If you do these things, how will it change the outcome?

_____

_____

_____

10. **Stop relapse quickly:** If you start eating compulsively/addictively, what can you do to stop?

_____

_____

_____

11. **Most important thing learned:** What is the most important thing you've learned by completing this exercise?

_____

_____

_____

Note: If you do relapse, it is important not to despair. You can chose to learn from the situation and find that in the future you can intervene before you eat compulsively/ addictively or experience life-damaging consequences. The important thing is that you learn to intervene as soon as you are able. For some people the recovery process seems to move steadily forward, but for many it goes forward, the person hits a stuck point, consolidates their resources, and then moves forward again. Whatever your recovery pattern is, you must not give up. Remember, recovery is a lifelong learning process.

> **This exercise stops here.**

Part 2: Mapping an Effectively Managed Situation

1. Think of a specific time when you experienced this high-risk situation and managed it in a way that you used effective recovery planning, and/or avoided eating compulsively/ addictively and adhered to your definition of abstinence. Tell the experience as if it were a story with a beginning, middle, and ending. (Start with the phrase: ***The high-risk situation began when…*** " Continue step by step. Start describing each step with the words: ***The next thing that happened was…*** " End the story with a final statement starting with the words: ***What finally happened was…*** ")

The high-risk situation began when…

_____

_____

_____

_____

_____

_____

_____

_____

_____

_____

_____

2. What did you want to accomplish by managing this situation the way you did?

_____

_____

3. Did you get what you wanted by managing the situation in this way? If yes, was it worth the cost or negative consequences you experienced?

❏ Yes   ❏   No   ❏   Unsure   Please explain:

_____

_____

_____

4. On a scale of 1 to 10, what were your stress levels when you managed the situation this way? _____

5. **Doing something different:** Can you think of some things you could do differently to manage the situation to produce an even better outcome?

_____

_____

_____

_____

6. **Avoiding the situation:** What could you have done to responsibly avoid getting into this high-risk situation?

_____

_____

_____

If you avoided this situation, how would it have changed the outcome?

_____

_____

_____

7. **Decision point #1:** What could you have done differently near the beginning of the high-risk situation to produce a better outcome? (How could you have thought differently? managed your feelings differently? fought your self-destructive urges differently? acted or behaved differently? treated other people differently?)

_____

_____

_____

If you do these things, how will it change the outcome?

_____

_____

_____

8. **Decision point #2:** What can you do differently near the middle of the high-risk situation to produce a better outcome? (How could you have thought differently? managed your feelings and emotions differently? fought your self-destructive urges differently? acted or behaved differently? treated other people differently?)

_____

_____

_____

If you do these things, how will it change the outcome?

_____

_____

_____

9. **Decision point #3:** What can you do differently near the end of the high-risk situation to produce a better outcome? (How could you have thought differently? managed your feelings and emotions differently? fought your self-destructive urges differently? acted or behaved differently? treated other people differently?)

_____

_____

_____

If you do these things, how will it change the outcome?

_____

_____

_____

10. **Stop relapse quickly:** If you start noticing a high-risk situation, what can you do to stop it?

_____

_____

_____

11. **Most important thing learned:** What is the most important thing you've learned by completing this exercise?

_____

_____

_____

_____

_____

> **This exercise stops here.**

Part 3: Mapping a Future High-Risk Situation

1. Think of the most important high-risk situation you will be experiencing in the near future. Imagine yourself managing that situation in a way that will cause you to eat compulsively/addictively and/or use ineffective recovery planning. Imagine yourself doing the things that you would have done in the past to convince yourself that it's OK to eat compulsively/addictively. Most people don't like this exercise, because it forces them to see what could happen if they do go back to self-defeating behaviors. Describe that experience as if it were a story with a beginning, middle, and ending.

    The high-risk situation will be triggered when...

    _____

    _____

    _____

    _____

    _____

    _____

    _____

    _____

    _____

    _____

    _____

2. What will you want to accomplish by managing the situation this way?

_____

_____

_____

3. Will you get what you want by managing it this way? If yes, will it be worth the cost or negative consequences you would experience?

❑ Yes   ❑   No   ❑   Unsure   Please explain:

_____

_____

_____

4. On a scale of 1 to 10, what will your stress levels be when you manage the situation this way? _____

5. Can you think of some things you could do differently to manage the situation without having to eat compulsively/addictively?

_____

_____

_____

6. **Avoiding the situation:** What can you do to responsibly avoid getting into this situation?

_____

_____

_____

If you avoid this situation, how will it change the outcome?

_____

_____

_____

7. **Decision point #1**: What can you do differently near the beginning of the situation to produce a better outcome? (How can you think differently? manage your feelings and emotions differently? fight your self-destructive urges differently? act or behave differently? treat other people differently?)

_____

If you do these things, how will it change the outcome?

_____

_____

_____

8. **Decision point #2:** What can you do differently near the middle of the situation to produce a better outcome? (How can you think differently? manage your feelings and emotions differently? fight your self-destructive urges differently? act or behave differently? treat other people differently?)

_____

_____

_____

If you do these things, how will it change the outcome?

_____

_____

_____

9. **Decision point #3:** What can you do differently near the end of the situation to produce a better outcome? (How can you think differently? manage your feelings and emotions differently? fight your self-destructive urges differently? act or behave differently? treat other people differently?)

_____

_____

If you do these things, how will it change the outcome?

_____

_____

_____

10. **Most important thing learned:** What is the most important thing you've learned by completing this exercise?

_____

_____

11. **Other future high-risk situations:** Are there other high-risk situations coming up in the near future that will put you at risk of eating compulsively/addictively?

❑ Yes   ❑   No   ❑   Unsure   Please describe them.

_____

_____

12. **Application to other high-risk situations:** How can you apply what you've learned in this situation to these other high-risk situations?

_____

_____

• At this point please go back to your intervention plan from *Exercise Five* and with what you have learned from this exercise, please fine-tune your plan.

Go to the next page and complete
the Situation Mapping Summary.

Part 4: Situation Mapping Summary

INSTRUCTIONS: Before your next group or individual session, take a few minutes to complete the following discussion questions and be prepared to share (not read) your reactions to the previous exercise.

1. As I was completing the exercises, I was thinking:

    _____

    _____

    _____

2. As I was completing the exercises, I was feeling:

    _____

    _____

    _____

3. What were the three situations you mapped and why did you pick those three?

    _____

    _____

    _____

4. The most important thing I learned as a result of completing this exercise was:

    _____

    _____

    _____

5. What I will do differently as a result of completing this exercise is:

    _____

    _____

    _____

This exercise stops here.

Exercise 9: Managing High-Risk Situations

High-risk situations, such as the ones that you mapped out in the previous exercise, can activate deeply entrenched habits of thinking, feeling, acting, and relating to others that make us want to eat compulsively/addictively or use other self-defeating behaviors. To effectively manage these high-risk situations we must learn to understand and control the way we react in these situations. Our chances of managing high-risk situations without eating compulsively/addictively or deviating from our definition of abstinence goes up as we get better at recognizing and managing our thoughts, feelings, urges, actions, and social reactions that make us want to eat compulsively/addictively.

Let's define some concepts that will help you to understand the process of learning how to manage your reactions to high-risk situations.

Personal reactions are automatic habitual things we do when something happens. There are four things we automatically do when something happens to us: we think about it, we have feelings or emotional reactions to it, we get an urge to do something about it, and we actually do something. So each automatic personal reaction can be broken down into its component parts: (1) automatic thoughts, (2) automatic feelings, (3) automatic urges, and (4) automatic actions. To learn how to effectively manage high-risk situations you must learn how to change automatic reactions into conscious choices.

Personal responses are different from personal reactions. A personal reaction is automatic and unconscious. A response is something we consciously choose to do. A conscious response is a choice. In order to manage high-risk situations without eating compulsively/addictively we must learn to make better choices about how to respond to the situation. In other words, to change automatic reactions into conscious choices we must choose what we think, how we manage and express our feelings, how we manage our urges, and what we actually do in these situations.

Addictive thinking is an irrational way of thinking that convinces people that eating compulsively/addictively is an effective way to manage the pain and problems caused by irresponsible thinking and behavior.

Irresponsible thinking is an irrational way of thinking about something that causes unnecessary emotional pain and motivates us to do things that will make our problems worse.

Addictive behavior is a way of acting that puts us around people, places, and things that make us want to eat compulsively/addictively.

Irresponsible behavior is a way of acting out or behaving that causes unnecessary pain and problems and may lead us to use other self-defeating behaviors.

There are *emotional consequences to thoughts and actions*. All thoughts and behaviors have logical consequences. Rational thinking allows people to deal with life without experiencing unnecessary emotional pain or the urge to eat compulsively/addictively to manage unpleasant feelings. Responsible behavior allows people to conduct their lives and solve their problems without producing unnecessary complications for themselves or others and without having to center their lives around eating.

Instant gratification is the desire to feel better now even if it means you will hurt worse in the future. A person seeking instant gratification wants to do something—anything—that will instantly make them feel better: *They want to feel better now without having to think better or act better first.* This results in a *quick-fix mentality*. People seeking instant gratification want to feel good all of the time. They tend to place feeling good above all other priorities. This is often based on the mistaken belief that if I feel better, I will be better, and my life will be better. They are not interested in living according to a responsible set of principles that will make their lives work well. They want what they want, when they want it, and how they want it, regardless of the consequences.

Deferred gratification is the ability to feel uncomfortable or to hurt now in order to gain a benefit or feel better in the future. People who use deferred gratification *think and act better first in order to feel better later*. To learn how to develop deferred gratification we must get in the habit of *thinking things through before we act them out*. Deferred gratification is based on the belief that there are rules or principles that will make our lives work well in the long run and will give us a firm sense of meaning, purpose, and satisfaction that will allow us to get through the inevitable periods of pain, hard feelings, and frustration we all experience as a normal part of life and living.

We can learn how to *challenge addictive and irresponsible thoughts:* We must learn how to identify and challenge our addictive and irresponsible thoughts if we want to make responsible choices that will allow us to build an effective and satisfying way of life. The following way of thinking can help you to challenge the tendency to seek instant gratification: The healthy goal is to live a good life regardless of how it feels at the moment. Feelings change; effective principles don't. Responsible people live a life based on principles, not feelings. Instant gratification provides what looks like an easy way out. The problem is that this easy way out becomes a trap. Once trapped in a conditioned pattern of instant gratification, you will feel cravings when you attempt to break the pattern. But once the pattern is broken, the urges disappear—because the long-term beneficial consequences of responsible living kick in. New brain science suggests that this change is the result of new neurological networks being developed in the brain. The problem is the old networks never go away, and, under stress, they can once again take over—hijacking the brain.

In this exercise on *managing personal reaction to high-risk situations* we will learn how to analyze high-risk situations by identifying the thoughts, feelings, urges, actions, and social reactions that make us want to eat compulsively/addictively. Then we will learn how to manage them in a new and more effective way without eating compulsively/addictively.

The first thing we need to do is to understand how thoughts, feelings, urges, actions, and social reactions relate to one another. Here are some basic principles that can help us to understand how this works.

1. *Thoughts cause feelings.* Whenever we think about something, we automatically react by having a feeling or an emotion.

2. *Thoughts and feelings work together to cause urges.* Our way of thinking causes us to feel certain feelings. These feelings, in turn, reinforce the way we are thinking. These thoughts and feelings work together to create an urge to do something. An urge is a desire that may be rational or irrational. The irrational urge to eat compulsively/addictively, even though we know that it will hurt us, is also called *craving*. It is irrational because we want to eat compulsively/addictively even though we know it will not be good for us.

3. *Urges plus decisions cause actions.* A decision is a choice. A choice is a specific way of thinking that causes us to commit to one way of doing things while refusing to do anything else. The space between the urge and the action is always filled with a decision. This decision may be an automatic and unconscious choice you have learned to make without having to think about it, or it can be based upon a conscious choice that results from carefully reflecting on the situation and the options available for dealing with it.

4. *Actions cause reactions from other people.* Our actions affect other people and cause them to react to us. It is helpful to think about our behavior like invitations we give to

63

other people to treat us in certain ways. Some behaviors invite people to be nice to us and to treat us with respect. Other behaviors invite people to argue and fight with us or to put us down. In every social situation we share a part of the responsibility for what happens, because we are constantly inviting people to respond to us by the actions we take and how we react to what other people do.

> • **Thoughts Cause Feelings**
>
> • **Thoughts and Feelings Cause Urges**
>
> • **Urges Plus Decisions Cause Actions**
>
> • **Actions Cause Social Reactions**

People who relapse usually have one or more of the following problems:

1. *They can't tell the difference between thoughts and feelings.* They tend to believe they can think anything they want and it won't affect their feelings. Then when they start to feel bad, they can't understand why and convince themselves that the only way to feel better is to eat compulsively/addictively.

2. *They can't tell the difference between feelings and urges.* They believe each feeling carries with it a specific urge. They don't realize they can experience a feeling, sit still and breath into the feeling and it will go away without being acted out.

3. *They can't tell the difference between urges and actions.* They don't realize there is a space between urge and action.

4. *They can't control their impulses.* They believe they must do whatever they feel an urge to do. They have never learned that to practice impulse control they must learn how to pause, relax, reflect, and decide—even though they feel a strong urge to act immediately. Let's look at the following four steps of the impulse control process:

   - *Pause* and notice the urge without doing anything about it.

   - *Relax* by taking a deep breath, slowly exhaling and consciously imagining the stress draining from your body.

   - *Reflect* on what you are experiencing by asking yourself, "What do I have an urge to do? What has happened when I have done similar things in the past? What is likely to happen if I do that now?"

   - *Decide* what you are going to do about the urge. Make a conscious choice instead of acting out in an automatic, unconscious way. When making the choice about what you are going to do, remind yourself that you will be responsible for both the action that you choose to take and its consequences.

> **Remember: *Impulse control lives in the space between the urge and the action.***

5. *They can't tell the difference between actions and social reactions.* They tend to believe that people respond to them for no reason at all. They don't link the responses of others to what they do when they are with others. In reality, what we do gives an invitation to other people to treat us in certain ways. Ask yourself, "How do I want to invite other people to treat me in this situation?"

With this in mind, let's complete an exercise that can help you identify and change the thoughts, feelings, urges, actions, and social reactions that can lead you back to compulsive/addictive eating.

> **Go to Part 1 to learn how to manage
> the thoughts related to this high-risk situation.**

Part 1: Managing Thoughts

In order to manage high-risk situations, we must learn how to identify the thoughts that can make us want to eat compulsively/addictively. Think of the high-risk situation you want to learn how to manage without using eating compulsively/addictively.

1. Go back to *Exercise 7, Part 1: Identifying High-Risk Situations* and write the title and the description of the high-risk situation you will be facing in the near future in the spaces below:

   Title of the High-Risk Situation: _____

   Description of the High-Risk Situation: *I know that I'm in a high-risk situation when*

   _____

   _____

   _____

2. Keeping the situation you described above in mind, read each of the thoughts listed below. Ask yourself if you tend to think similar thoughts when you are in this high-risk situation. If you do, put a check in the box in front of the thought. Check as many boxes as you need to.

   ❑ A. I have a right to eat any way I want, and nobody has the right to tell me to stop.
   ❑ B. I don't have problems because of eating. I eat to cope with problems.
   ❑ C. I do have problems with eating or abstinence, but they're not that bad.
   ❑ D. I have eating problems, but I have a good reason for having them!
   ❑ E. I have eating or abstinence problems, but they're not my fault!
   ❑ F. I always feel good and never feel bad or have problems when I'm eating *my* way.
   ❑ G. Eating can magically fix me and solve my problems.
   ❑ H. Eating is good for me and lets me feel good and have a better quality of life.
   ❑ I. Eating *my* way lets me do things that I can't do otherwise.
   ❑ J. Eating lets me handle pain and solve problems I couldn't manage otherwise.
   ❑ K. Eating *my* way makes it easy for me to deal with people and build relationships.
   ❑ L. I am in control of my eating and abstinence; it does not control me.
   ❑ M. I must control my eating and abstinence or I will be no good.

> **Go to the next page to list your specific needs.**

65

3. What are the three thoughts you tend to have in this kind of high-risk situation that make you want to eat compulsively/addictively? You can use the thoughts above as a starting point, but it is important for you to put these thoughts in your own words. Please don't censor them.

Thought #1: _____

_____

What is another way of thinking that could convince you not to eat compulsively/addictively?

_____

_____

Thought #2: _____

_____

What is another way of thinking that could convince you not to eat compulsively/addictively?

_____

_____

Thought #3: _____

_____

What is another way of thinking that could convince you not to eat compulsively/addictively?

_____

_____

> **Go to Part 2 to learn how to manage
> the feelings related to this high-risk situation.**

Part 2: Managing Feelings

The following exercise will show you how to more effectively manage the feelings and emotions you will tend to experience in your immediate high-risk situation that could lead to eating compulsively/addictively or deviating from your personal definition of abstinence.

Before completing this part of the exercise, go back and read the title and the description of the high-risk situation you are learning how to manage.

1. When you are in this high-risk situation, do you tend to feel...

   ❑ *Strong*   or   ❑ *Weak?*   How intense is the feeling? (0–10) _____

   Why do you rate it this way?_____

2. When you are in this high-risk situation, do you tend to feel...

   ❏ *Caring* or ❏ *Angry?* How intense is the feeling? (0–10) _____
   Why do you rate it this way? _____

3. When you are in this high-risk situation, do you tend to feel...

   ❏ *Happy* or ❏ *Sad?* How intense is the feeling? (0–10) _____
   Why do you rate it this way? _____

4. When you are in this high-risk situation, do you tend to feel...

   ❏ *Safe* or ❏ *Threatened?* How intense is the feeling? (0–10) _____
   Why do you rate it this way? _____

5. When you are in this high-risk situation, do you tend to feel...

   ❏ *Fulfilled* or ❏ *Frustrated?* How intense is the feeling? (0–10) _____
   Why do you rate it this way? _____

6. When you are in this high-risk situation, do you tend to feel...

   ❏ *Proud* or ❏ *Ashamed?* How intense is the feeling? (0–10) _____
   Why do you rate it this way? _____

7. When you are in this high-risk situation, do you tend to feel...

   ❏ *Connected* or ❏ *Lonely?* How intense is the feeling? (0–10) _____
   Why do you rate it this way? _____

8. When you are in this high-risk situation, do you tend to feel...

   ❏ *Peaceful* or ❏ *Agitated?* How intense is the feeling? (0–10) _____
   Why do you rate it this way? _____

9. What are the three strongest feelings you tend to have in this kind of high-risk situation that makes you want to eat compulsively/addictively?

   Feeling #1: _____
   Why did you choose this feeling? _____

   _____

   Feeling #2: _____
   Why did you choose this feeling? _____

   _____

   Feeling #3: _____
   Why did you choose this feeling? _____

   _____

10. Keeping these three feelings in mind, read each of the following statements about your ability to manage your feelings and rate how true it is on a scale of 0–10. ("0" means the statement is not at all true; "10" means the statement is totally true.) Place your answer on the line in front of each statement.

___ **Skill #1:** I am able to anticipate situations that are likely to provoke strong feelings and emotions.

___ **Skill #2:** I am able to recognize when I am starting to have a strong feeling or emotion.

___ **Skill #3:** I am able to stop myself from automatically reacting to the feeling without thinking it through.

___ **Skill #4:** I am able to call a time-out in emotionally charged situations before my feelings become unmanageable.

___ **Skill #5:** I am able to use an immediate relaxation technique to bring down the intensity of the feeling.

___ **Skill #6:** I am able to take a deep breath and notice what I'm feeling.

___ **Skill #7:** I am able to find words that describe what I'm feeling and use the feeling list when necessary.

___ **Skill #8:** I am able to rate the intensity of my feelings using a ten-point scale.

___ **Skill #9:** I am able to consciously acknowledge the feeling and its intensity by saying to myself, "Right now I'm feeling _____ and it's OK to be feeling this way."

___ **Skill #10:** I am able to identify what I'm thinking that's making me feel this way and ask myself, "How can I change my thinking in a way that will make me feel better?"

___ **Skill #11:** I am able to identify what I'm doing that's making me feel this way and ask myself, "How can I change what I'm doing in a way that will make me feel better?"

___ **Skill #12:** I am able to recognize and resist urges to create problems, hurt myself, or hurt other people in an attempt to make myself feel better.

___ **Skill #13:** I am able to recognize my resistance to doing things that would help me or my situation, and force myself to do those things despite the resistance.

___ **Skill #14:** I am able to get outside of myself and recognize and respond to what other people are feeling.

Go to the next section to list *your* specific feelings.

11. **Strongest Feeling:** Review the three feelings you identified in question 9 on page 67. What is the strongest feeling you experience in this high-risk situation?

_____

A. What are you *thinking* that makes you feel this way?

_____

_____

B. What is another way of thinking that could make you feel different?

_____

_____

C. What are you doing that makes you feel this way?

_____

_____

D. What is another way of acting that could make you feel different?

_____

_____

12. **Second Strongest Feeling:** Review the three feelings you identified in question 9. What is the second strongest feeling you experience in this high-risk situation?

_____

A. What are you *thinking* that makes you feel this way?

_____

_____

B. What is another way of thinking that could make you feel different?

_____

_____

C. What are you doing that makes you feel this way?

_____

_____

D. What is another way of acting that could make you feel different?

_____

_____

13. **Third Strongest Feeling:** Review the three feelings you identified in question 9. What is the third strongest feeling you experience in this high-risk situation?

_____

A.   What are you *thinking* that makes you feel this way?

_____

_____

B.   What is another way of thinking that could make you feel different?

_____

_____

C.   What are you doing that makes you feel this way?

_____

_____

D.   What is another way of acting that could make you feel different?

_____

_____

> **Go to Part 3 to learn how to manage
> the urges related to this high-risk situation.**

Part 3: Managing Urges

High-risk situations often cause the urge to eat compulsively/addictively. When this urge or craving is activated, we almost always experience an inner conflict between two parts of ourselves. One part, our addictive self, wants us to eat compulsively/addictively or deviate from our personal definition of abstinence. Another part of us, the sober self, wants us to manage the situation without eating compulsively/addictively and adhere to our abstinence. This exercise will help you explore these two parts of yourself.

1.   Before completing this part of the exercise, go back and read the title and the description of the high-risk situation you are learning how to manage.

2.   When you are in this high-risk situation, what do you have an urge to do?

_____

_____

3.   Is there a part of you that wants to eat compulsively/addictively? Tell me about that part of you.

_____

_____

_____

4.   Is there another part of you that wants to manage the situation without eating compulsively/addictively? Tell me about that part of you.

70

_____

_____

_____

5. If you wanted to manage this high-risk situation more effectively, what part of you do you need to listen to and why?

_____

_____

_____

> **Go to Part 4 to learn how to manage
> the actions related to this high-risk situation.**

Part 4: Managing Actions/Behaviors

1. Before completing this part of the exercise, go back and read the title and the description of the high-risk situation you are learning how to manage.

2. Keeping this high-risk situation in mind, read the following list of *Self-Defeating Behaviors* that can be used to mismanage this high-risk situation. Check the behaviors you are most likely to use in this situation.

    ❑ A. **Procrastinating:** I put off dealing with the high-risk situation by finding excuses or reasons for not doing it now.

    ❑ B. **Distracting myself:** I get too busy with other things to pay attention to managing the situation.

    ❑ C. **Saying "It's not that important":** I convince myself that other things are more important than effectively managing this high-risk situation.

    ❑ D. **Thinking I'm cured:** I convince myself that because I'm OK now and don't have an eating problem anymore, there is no need to learn how to manage this high-risk situation more effectively.

    ❑ E. **Playing dumb:** Even though a big part of me knows what I need to do to manage this situation more effectively, I let myself get confused and convince myself and others that I can't understand what I'm supposed to do.

    ❑ F. **Getting overwhelmed:** I feel scared and start to panic. I use my fear as an excuse for not learning how to manage the high-risk situation more effectively.

    ❑ G. **Playing helpless:** I pretend to be too weak and helpless to manage the situation more effectively. Sometimes I can even convince myself that I am helpless.

    ❑ H. **Wanting the quick fix:** I want a guarantee that I can quickly and easily learn to manage the high-risk situation more effectively or I won't even try.

3. What are the three self-defeating behaviors you tend to have in this kind of high-risk situation that make you want to eat compulsively/addictively? You can use the self-defeating behaviors above as a starting point, but it is important for you to write the descriptions in your own words. You may have others that are not on this list.

71

A.   **Self-Defeating Behavior #1:**

_____

_____

What is another way of behaving that could stop you from eating compulsively/addictively in this situation?

_____

_____

B.   **Self-Defeating Behavior #2:**

_____

_____

What is another way of behaving that could stop you from eating compulsively/addictively in this situation?

_____

_____

C.   **Self-Defeating Behavior #3:**

_____

_____

What is another way of behaving that could stop you from eating compulsively/addictively in this situation?

_____

_____

4.   When you use these self-defeating behaviors…

A.   How do other people react to you in a way that increases your risk of eating compulsively/addictively?

_____

_____

B.   How could other people react to you in a way that would help you to stay away from eating compulsively/addictively?

_____

_____

C.   What could you do to invite other people to deal with you in a way that would help you to stay away from eating compulsively/addictively when you get into high-risk situations?

_____

_____

Go to Part 5 to tie together everything you have learned about managing this kind of situation.

Part 5: Tying It All Together

The fifth part of this exercise will help you tie together everything you have learned from completing Parts 1–4.

1. Before completing this part of the exercise, go back and read the title and the description of the high-risk situation you are learning how to manage. Then review your answers to all of the questions in Parts 1–4. Take time to reflect on what you are really saying in your answers. See if you can sense how the answer to each question is somehow connected to all of your other answers. Then complete the questions in the table below.

2. When you're in this high-risk situation, what do you tend to think?	2-a. What is another way of thinking that will allow you to manage this high-risk situation without eating compulsively/addictively?
_____ _____ _____ _____ _____ _____	_____ _____ _____ _____ _____ _____
3. When you're in this high-risk situation, what do you tend to feel?	3-a. What is another way to manage those feelings that will let you manage this situation without eating compulsively/addictively?
_____ _____ _____ _____ _____	_____ _____ _____ _____ _____

4. When you're in this high-risk situation, what do you have an urge to do?	4-a. What is another way of managing this urge that will allow you to manage this situation without eating compulsively/addictively?
_____ _____ _____ _____ _____ _____	_____ _____ _____ _____ _____
5. When you're in this high-risk situation, what do you usually do?	5-a. What are some other things that you could do that would allow you to manage this situation without eating compulsively/addictively?
_____ _____ _____ _____ _____	_____ _____ _____ _____ _____
6. When you're in this high-risk situation, how do other people usually react?	6-a. How could you invite other people to react to you in a way that would help you manage this situation without eating compulsively/addictively?
_____ _____ _____ _____ _____	_____ _____ _____ _____ _____

7. **Most Important Thing Learned:** What is the most important thing you've learned by completing this exercise?

_____

_____

_____

_____

_____

_____

_____

_____

**Go to the next page and complete
the High-Risk Situation Management Summary.**

Part 6: High-Risk Situation Management Summary

INSTRUCTIONS: Before your next group or individual session, take a few minutes to complete the following discussion questions and be prepared to share (not read) your reactions to the previous exercises.

1. As I was completing the exercises, I was thinking:

   _____

   _____

   _____

2. As I was completing the exercises, I was feeling:

   _____

   _____

   _____

3. What were the most problematic thoughts, feelings, and behaviors you identified? Why did you choose those specific items, and what were your management strategies?

   _____

   _____

   _____

4. The most important thing I learned as a result of completing this exercise was:

   _____

   _____

   _____

5. What I plan to do differently as a result of completing this exercise is:

   _____

   _____

   _____

   _____

   _____

   _____

   ┌───┐

   This exercise stops here.

   └───┘

Exercise 10: Recovery Planning

Part 1: Selecting Recovery Activities

Having a plan for each day will help you recover with practicing better eating management, adhering to your personal definition of abstinence, and following your Healthy Living Plan. People who successfully recover tend to do certain basic things. These recovery principles are proven. In AA (Alcoholics Anonymous), there is such a strong belief in them that many people with solid recovery will say, "If you want what we have, do what we did!" and, "It works if you work it!" The same applies to those recovering from compulsive/addictive eating. They have learned to develop a recovery/management plan. However, not everyone does exactly the same things. Once you understand yourself and the basic principles of recovery, abstinence, a Healthy Living Plan, and relapse prevention, you can build an effective personal program for yourself.

When people first read the following list, they tend to get defensive. "I can't do all of those things!" they say to themselves. We invite you to think about your recovery as if you were hiking in the Grand Canyon and had to jump across a ravine that's about three feet wide and 100 feet deep. It's better to jump three feet too far than to risk jumping one inch too short. The same is true of recovery. It's better to plan to do a little bit more than you need to do than to risk not doing enough. In AA they say, "Half measures availed us nothing!"

The seven basic recovery activities described below are actually habits of good, healthy living. Anyone who wants to live a responsible, healthy, and fulfilling life will get in the habit of regularly doing these things. For people in any type of recovery, these activities are essential, and if you are recovering from a compulsive/addictive eating condition, these steps become even more crucial. A regular schedule of these activities—designed to match your unique profile of recovery needs, eating management requirements, and high-risk situations—is necessary for your brain and body to heal from the damage caused by compulsively/addictively eating.

Instructions: Read the list of recovery activities that follow, and identify which activities you think will be helpful for your recovery and eating management program. Notice the obstacles you face in doing them on a regular basis, and indicate your strategies to overcome these obstacles.

Go to the next page and complete the Selecting Recovery Activities.

1. **Professional Counseling:** The success of your recovery and effective eating management will depend on regular attendance at education sessions, group therapy sessions, and individual therapy sessions. The scientific literature on treatment effectiveness clearly shows that the more time you invest in professional counseling and therapy during the first two years of recovery, the more likely you are to stay in recovery. This process needs to include eating management treatment planning. There are now professionals across the United States and in other countries that specialize in the treatment of eating disorders. Ask any potential counselor, therapist, or psychiatrist about their qualifications before getting involved in a therapeutic relationship.

   A. Do I believe that I need to do this? ❑ Yes ❑ No ❑ Unsure
   Please explain:

   _____

   _____

   B. The obstacles that might prevent me from doing this are:

   _____

   _____

   C. Possible ways of overcoming these obstacles are:

   _____

   _____

   D. Will I put this on my recovery plan? ❑ Yes ❑ No ❑ Unsure
   Please explain:

   _____

   _____

2. **Self-Help Programs:** There are a number of self-help programs that can support you in your efforts to live a sober and responsible life, such as Overeaters Anonymous (OA) and Eating Disorders Anonymous (EDA). Some people with food issues have found Rational Recovery (or SMART Recovery) helpful. These programs all have several things in common: (1) They ask you to abstain from compulsive/addictive eating patterns and to live a responsible life; (2) they encourage you to regularly attend meetings so you can meet and develop relationships with other people living sober and responsible lives; (3) they ask you to meet regularly with an established member of the group (usually called a sponsor) who will help you learn about the organization and get through the rough spots; and (4) they promote a program of recovery (often in the form of steps or structured exercises for you to work on outside of meetings) that focuses on techniques for changing your thinking, emotional management, urge management, and behavior.

   Scientific research shows that the more committed and actively involved you are in self-help groups during the first two years of recovery, the greater your ability to avoid relapse. You should also consider joining an appropriate eating support group because research indicates that personal empowerment is crucial for developing effective, long-term eating management. Potential groups for you can be found at *www.dietingrecov ery.com*.

One note of caution as you begin attending Twelve-Step meetings: While these meetings are *crucial* for your recovery, it is very important that the group you attend does not attempt to define your meal planning for you. That plan is determined with you and your medical provider, nutritionist, or registered dietician. If you begin attending a particular group and they suggest that you delete an entire food group from your plan of eating or you *must* eat a particular food at a specific time of day, we encourage you to find a different group.

We believe it is crucial to add a note about sponsorship: The relationship with a sponsor can be a terrific support and growth opportunity. However, it is equally important that you get a sense that the person you ask to sponsor you has stable recovery for an extended period of time (ideally longer than a year) and is not engaging in dieting disguised as twelfth-step fellowship. For example, being slim is not the hallmark you want to look for in a sponsor. Your impression of what slim and healthy is may be quite skewed at this point in your illness. Many eating addicts never become overweight—even in the height of their illness—so that benchmark may not be accurate.

What you can look for is a person who seems generally emotionally stable, discusses having a stable plan of eating, and has worked the Twelve Steps straight through at least once. Again, the relationship with a sponsor can be a unique and wonderfully supportive experience; we encourage you to choose wisely.

A. Do I believe that I need to do this? ❑ Yes ❑ No ❑ Unsure
   Please explain:

   _____

   _____

B. The obstacles that might prevent me from doing this are:

   _____

   _____

C. Possible ways of overcoming these obstacles are:

   _____

   _____

D. Will I put this on my recovery plan? ❑ Yes ❑ No ❑ Unsure
   Please explain:

   _____

   _____

3. **Proper Nutrition:** What you eat can affect how you think, feel, and act. Recovering people find they feel better if they eat three well-balanced meals a day; others need more. Your nutrition plan should be developed with an appropriate medical provider or nutritionist who might suggest using vitamin and amino acid supplements, avoiding eating sugar and foods made with white flour, cutting back or stopping cigarette smoking and the drinking of beverages containing caffeine, such as coffee and colas. Recovering people who don't follow these simple principles of healthy diet and meal planning tend

to feel anxious and depressed, have strong and violent mood swings, feel constantly angry and resentful, and periodically experience powerful cravings. They're more likely to relapse. Those who follow a nutritious eating plan 60–80 percent of the time tend to feel better and have lower relapse rates. Proper nutrition is crucial for effective eating management.

A. Do I believe that I need to do this?　❑　Yes　❑　No　❑　Unsure
Please explain:

_____

_____

B. The obstacles that might prevent me from doing this are:

_____

_____

C. Possible ways of overcoming these obstacles are:

_____

_____

D. Will I put this on my recovery plan?　❑　Yes　❑　No　❑　Unsure
Please explain:

_____

_____

4. **Exercise Program:** If your physical condition permits, doing thirty minutes of aerobic exercise each day will help your brain recover and help you feel better about yourself. Fast walking, jogging, swimming, and aerobics classes are all helpful. It's also helpful to do strength-building exercises (such as weight lifting) and flexibility exercises (such as stretching) in addition to the aerobic exercise. You need to work with your doctor or healthcare practitioner to determine the most effective (and safest) exercise program for you.

A. Do I believe that I need to do this?　❑　Yes　❑　No　❑　Unsure
Please explain:

_____

_____

B. The obstacles that might prevent me from doing this are:

_____

_____

C. Possible ways of overcoming these obstacles are:

_____

_____

D. Will I put this on my recovery plan?　❑　Yes　❑　No　❑　Unsure
Please explain:

_____

_____

5. **Stress Management Program:** Stress is a major cause of relapse. In addition, an increase in stress often leads to an increase in cravings to eat compulsively/addictively. Recovering people who learn how to manage stress without using self-defeating behaviors tend to stay in recovery and learn how to more effectively manage their relapse triggers. Those who don't learn to manage stress tend to relapse or suffer more. Stress management involves learning relaxation exercises and taking quiet time on a daily basis to relax. It also involves avoiding long hours of working and taking time for recreation and relaxation. Meditation can also be part of this program.

A. Do I believe that I need to do this?　❑　Yes　❑　No　❑　Unsure
Please explain:

_____

_____

B. The obstacles that might prevent me from doing this are:

_____

_____

C. Possible ways of overcoming these obstacles are:

_____

_____

D. Will I put this on my recovery plan?　❑　Yes　❑　No　❑　Unsure
Please explain:

_____

_____

6. **Spiritual Development Program:** Human beings have both a physical self (based on the health of their brains and bodies) and a nonphysical self (based on the health of their value systems and spiritual lives). Most recovering people find they need to invest regular time in developing themselves spiritually (in other words, exercising the nonphysical aspects of who they are). Twelve-Step programs such as OA provide an excellent

program for spiritual recovery, as do many communities of faith and spiritual programs. At the heart of any spiritual program are three activities: (1) fellowship, during which you spend time talking with other people who use similar methods; (2) private prayer and meditation, during which you take time alone to be conscious of yourself in the presence of your Higher Power or to consciously reflect upon your spiritual self; and (3) group worship, during which you pray and meditate with other people who share a similar spiritual philosophy.

A. Do I believe that I need to do this?　❑　Yes　❑　No　❑　Unsure
Please explain:

_____

_____

B. The obstacles that might prevent me from doing this are:

_____

_____

C. Possible ways of overcoming these obstacles are:

_____

_____

D. Will I put this on my recovery plan?　❑　Yes　❑　No　❑ Unsure
Please explain:

_____

_____

7. **Morning and Evening Inventories:** People who avoid relapse and successfully obtain lifelong recovery learn how to break free of automatic and unconscious self-defeating responses. They learn to live consciously each day, being aware of what they're doing and taking responsibility for what they do and its consequences. To stay consciously aware, they take time each morning to plan their day (a morning planning inventory), and they take time each evening to review their progress and problems (an evening review inventory). They discuss what they learn about themselves with other people who are involved in their recovery program.

For people with compulsive eating problems, keeping a journal of their emotions helps to identify stress and trigger patterns as well as associated thoughts, feelings, and behaviors. During times of increased stress, keeping a daily journal is essential, leading to more effective eating management.

A. Do I believe that I need to do this?　❑　Yes　❑　No　❑　Unsure
Please explain:

_____

_____

B. The obstacles that might prevent me from doing this are:

_____

_____

C. Possible ways of overcoming these obstacles are:

_____

_____

D. Will I put this on my recovery plan? ❑ Yes ❑ No ❑ Unsure
   Please explain:

_____

_____

**Go to the next page and complete
The Schedule of Recovery Activities.**

Part 2: The Schedule of Recovery Activities

INSTRUCTIONS: On the next page is a weekly planner that will allow you to create a schedule of weekly recovery and eating-management activities. Think of a typical week and enter the eating-management and recovery activities that you plan to routinely schedule in the correct time slot for each day. *Recovery activities* and/or *eating management activities* are specific things you do at scheduled times on certain days. If you can't enter the activity onto a daily planner at a specific time, it's not a recovery and/or eating-management activity. Most people find it crucial to have more than one scheduled activity for each day.

**Go to the next page and build
a weekly schedule of recovery activities.**

Weekly Planner

	Sunday	Monday	Tuesday	Wednesday	Thursday	Friday	Saturday
6:00 AM							
6:30 AM							
7:00 AM							
7:30 AM							
8:00 AM							
8:30 AM							
9:00 AM							
9:30 AM							
10:00 AM							
10:30 AM							
11:00 AM							
11:30 AM							
12:00 Noon							
12:30 PM							
1:00 PM							
1:30 PM							
2:00 PM							
2:30 PM							
3:00 PM							
3:30 PM							
4:00 PM							
4:30 PM							
5:00 PM							
5:30 PM							
6:00 PM							
6:30 PM							
7:00 PM							
7:30 PM							
8:00 PM							
8:30 PM							
9:00 PM							
9:30 PM							
10:00 PM							
10:30 PM							

Go to the next page and complete the Testing the Schedule of Recovery Activities exercise.

Part 3: Testing the Schedule of Recovery Activities

INSTRUCTIONS:

1. Go back to *Exercise 7-1, Identifying High-Risk Situations*, and review the primary high-risk situation that you want your recovery and eating-management program to help you identify and manage. Read the personal title and description and the thought, feeling, urge, and action statements carefully. What is the personal title and description of this high-risk situation?

   Title:_____

   Description: *I know that I'm in a high-risk situation when...*

   _____

   _____

2. Review your weekly planner. What is the most important recovery and/or eating management activity that will help you manage this high-risk situation?

   _____

   _____

   A. How can you use this recovery and/or eating-management activity to help you identify this high-risk situation should it occur? (Remember, most high-risk situations develop in an automatic and unconscious way. A trigger is activated, and we start using the old ways of thinking and acting without being consciously aware of what we're doing. To prevent relapse it's helpful to regularly schedule recovery and/or eating management activities that will encourage us to talk about how we're thinking, feeling, and acting, and then receive feedback if we experience high-risk situations.)

      _____

      _____

   B. If you start to experience this high-risk situation again, how can you use this recovery activity to manage it? (Remember, managing a high-risk situation means changing how you think, feel, and act. How can this recovery activity help you stop thinking and doing things that make you feel like relapsing? How can it help you start thinking and doing things that make you want to get back into recovery?)

      _____

      _____

3. Review your weekly planner again. What is the second most important recovery activity that will help you manage this high-risk situation?

   _____

   _____

   A. How can you use this recovery activity to help you identify this high-risk situation?

      _____

      _____

86

B. If you start to experience this high-risk situation again, how can you use this recovery activity to manage it?

_____

_____

4. Review your weekly planner one last time. What is the third most important recovery activity that will help you manage this high-risk situation?

_____

_____

A. How can you use this recovery activity to help you identify this high-risk situation should it occur?

_____

_____

B. If you start to experience this high-risk situation again, how can you use this recovery activity to manage it?

_____

_____

5. What other recovery activities can you think of that could be more effective in helping you identify and manage this high-risk situation should it occur?

_____

_____

At this point we suggest you go back to your Relapse Intervention Plan in *Exercise Five* and fine-tune it one final time before going to the Recovery Planning Summary. This is also a plan you might want to review at least once a month for the first year of your recovery process.

**Go to the next page and complete
the Recovery Planning Summary.**

Part 4: Recovery Planning Summary

INSTRUCTIONS: Before your next group or individual session take a few minutes to complete the following discussion questions and be prepared to share (not read) your reactions to the previous exercise.

1. As I was completing the exercises, I was thinking:

   _____

   _____

2. As I was completing the exercises, I was feeling:

   _____

   _____

3. What were the most important recovery activities you scheduled, and why did you choose those specific activities? How will they help you manage your high-risk situations?

   _____

   _____

   _____

   _____

   _____

4. The most important thing I learned as a result of completing this exercise was:

   _____

   _____

   _____

   _____

5. What I plan to do differently as a result of completing this exercise is:

   _____

   _____

   _____

   _____

This exercise stops here.

88

Exercise 11: Final Evaluation

INSTRUCTIONS: The ultimate test of whether you have benefited from completing the exercises in this workbook will be your ability to increase effective eating management, follow your Healthy Living Plan, adhere to your personal definition of abstinence, and avoid relapse. It may be helpful, however, to review what you have accomplished. A careful evaluation may help you identify areas in your Relapse Prevention Plan that are incomplete. By going back and completing these areas, you may avoid unnecessary relapse and the resulting pain and problems.

Here is a checklist that can help you decide if you have accomplished the objectives of completing this workbook. Read each statement and ask yourself if you have fully completed that objective, partially completed it, or not completed it at all. *Remember:* This is a self-evaluation designed to help you determine if you have the skills needed to avoid relapse. Be honest with yourself. If you relapse because you haven't learned the necessary skills to stay in recovery, you are the one who will pay the price.

1. *Healthy Living Planning:* I understand and can explain the principles of a Healthy Living Plan and can develop my own personal Biopsychosocialspiritual Healthy Living Plan.

   Level of Completion: ❑ None (0) ❑ Partial (5) ❑ Full (10) *Score (0–10):* _____

2. *Creating Your Definition of Abstinence:* I have now personalized and articulated my own personal understanding of abstinence by completing this exercise.

   Level of Completion: ❑ None (0) ❑ Partial (5) ❑ Full (10) *Score (0–10):* _____

3. *The Eating Addiction Problem Checklist:* I can use the *Eating Addiction Problem Checklist* to honestly assess my personal level of problems with eating.

   Level of Completion: ❑ None (0) ❑ Partial (5) ❑ Full (10) *Score (0–10):* _____

4. *Decision Making about Eating Addiction:* I understand and can explain the reasons why I started eating compulsively/addictively. I understand and can explain the reasons why I stopped eating problematically, as well as what I did to stay abstinent.

   Level of Completion: ❑ None (0) ❑ Partial (5) ❑ Full (10) *Score (0–10):* _____

5. *Healthy Living Contract Intervention Planning:* I can define what my Healthy Living Plan and recovery plan include. I have completed and signed a healthy living contract, agreeing to maintain my Healthy Living Plan and effective eating management.

   Level of Completion: ❑ None (0) ❑ Partial (5) ❑ Full (10) *Score (0–10):* _____

6. *Identifying High-Risk Situations:* I am able to identify the immediate high-risk situations that can cause me to eat compulsively/addictively and/or stop using an effective food management program despite my commitment not to by developing an *Initial High-Risk Situation List* and identifying my immediate high-risk situations.

   Level of Completion: ❑ None (0) ❑ Partial (5) ❑ Full (10) *Score (0–10):* _____

7. *Personalizing High-Risk Situations:* I am able to concretely and specifically describe the immediate high-risk situations, having developed meaningful

   - personal titles and
   - personal descriptions.

Level of Completion: ❑ None (0) ❑ Partial (5) ❑ Full (10) *Score (0–10):* _____

8. ***Mapping Past Mismanaged High-Risk Situations:*** I am able to use *Situation Mapping* to objectively describe past high-risk situations that were managed in a way that led to eating compulsively/addictively.

   Level of Completion: ❑ None (0) ❑ Partial (5) ❑ Full (10) *Score (0–10):* _____

9. ***Analyzing Past Mismanaged High-Risk Situations:*** I am able to use *High-Risk Situation Analysis* to identify the thoughts, feelings, urges, actions, and relationship patterns caused by the past mismanagement of the high-risk situation.

   Level of Completion: ❑ None (0) ❑ Partial (5) ❑ Full (10) *Score (0–10):* _____

10. ***Managing High-Risk Thoughts and Feelings:*** I am able to: (1) identify the general way of thinking that is driving situational mismanagement; (2) show the relationship between these thoughts and the feelings driving mismanagement; and (3) use positive self-talk techniques to challenge the thoughts and feelings driving situational mismanagement.

    Level of Completion: ❑ None (0) ❑ Partial (5) ❑ Full (10) *Score (0–10):* _____

11. ***Mapping Future High-Risk Situations:*** I can identify and map future high-risk situations, identify similar past situations that were managed without eating compulsively/addictively, identify the critical intervention points in those situations, and use new thoughts and behaviors that will allow me to manage the situation by using an appropriate eating-management plan and/or avoid eating compulsively/addictively.

    Level of Completion: ❑ None (0) ❑ Partial (5) ❑ Full (10) *Score (0–10):* _____

12. ***Developing a Recovery Plan:*** I am able to develop a schedule of recovery activities that will support my ongoing identification and management of high-risk situations and help me to intervene early should returning to compulsive/addictive eating (relapse) occur.

    Level of Completion: ❑ None (0) ❑ Partial (5) ❑ Full (10) *Score (0–10):* _____

13. ***Overall Skill Level:*** I have developed an overall ability to identify and manage my high-risk situations that lead me from stable recovery to relapse and have developed a schedule of recovery activities that will support my ongoing high-risk situation identification and management.

    Level of Completion: ❑ None (0) ❑ Partial (5) ❑ Full (10) *Score (0–10):* _____

If you identified any areas where you feel you need more work, let your counselor, sponsor, or appropriate support person know. Remember, it's best to be completely prepared to manage the high-risk situations that can lead to relapse and/or compulsive/addictive eating.

> **This exercise stops here. Go to the next page.**
> **We have some final words to share with you.**

A Final Word

Congratulations! You now belong to a growing group of recovering people who have invested time and energy to learn how to identify and manage their high-risk situations. The clinical exercises that you learned by completing this workbook and the *Healthy Living Plan* you developed can be used immediately to help you to identify and manage the high-risk situations that cause relapse. Hopefully you will have internalized a system of problem solving that can be applied to many problems you will experience in your recovery.

The challenge of recovery is never really over. It seems that once we start a recovery process, we are either growing or we're dying. There is no standing still. We either commit ourselves each day to improving and refining our recovery skills, or we become complacent and slowly move toward meaninglessness, misery, and relapse. We must make a conscious choice each day about which path we'll follow. The recovery process can be compared to walking up a down escalator. If you stand still, you go down (AKA relapse).

As you move from completing this workbook to using your new skills in real-life situations, remember that temporary setbacks may occur. But you can always choose to go back to your recovery process. *Recovery is possible.* By completing this workbook you have already taken a big step toward improving your recovery and lowering your risk of relapse. Your next job is to use the skills that you have learned in your day-to-day life.

Remember, if you get stuck anywhere in the process of identifying and managing high-risk situations, you can go to our Web site at *www.cenaps.com* and check out our list of certified relapse prevention specialists to contact for additional support. You can also send an e-mail to *info@cenaps.com* to ask a question or have someone get back to you.

> **Good luck on your journey of effective eating management and your recovery! We're pleased and proud to have walked with you for a little while along the way. Thank you for permitting us to do so!**

—*Dr. Stephen F. Grinstead and Dr. Shari Stillman-Corbitt*

Notes